DATE DUE

.C. 38-2931

Read My Lips

A Complete Guide to the Vagina and Vulva

Debby Herbenick, PhD
and
Vanessa Schick, PhD

ROWMAN & LITTLEFIELD PUBLISHERS, INC.
Lanham • Boulder • New York • Toronto • Plymouth, UK

Published by Rowman & Littlefield Publishers, Inc.
A wholly owned subsidiary of The Rowman & Littlefield Publishing Group, Inc.
4501 Forbes Boulevard, Suite 200, Lanham, Maryland 20706
http://www.rowmanlittlefield.com

Estover Road, Plymouth PL6 7PY, United Kingdom

Distributed by NATIONAL BOOK NETWORK

British Library Cataloguing in Publication Information Available

Library of Congress Cataloging-in-Publication Data

Herbenick, Debby.
    Read my lips : a complete guide to the vagina and vulva / Debby Herbenick
and Vanessa Schick.
        p.   cm.
    Includes bibliographical references and index.
    ISBN 978-1-4422-0800-1 (pbk.) — ISBN 978-1-4422-0802-5 (electronic)
    1. Vulva—Popular works.   2. Vagina—Popular works.   3. Women—
Health and hygiene—Popular works.   I. Schick, Vanessa, 1982–   II. Title.

RG268.H47 2011
612.6'28—dc23

                                                                2011019793

This book is dedicated to the many men and women whose stories have inspired us to think about vulvas and vaginas in complex and intricate ways.
We hope that *Read My Lips* will do the same for some of you.

Contents

Acknowledgments

$\mathcal{W}$e would like to thank our editor, Suzanne Staszak-Silva, for helping to turn our quirky book filled with crafts and puns into a reality. Thank you for your patience and your confidence in our work. We are enormously grateful to our fantastic agent, Kate Lee, whose advice and encouragement were instrumental. Of course, no matter how many words we used, a description of a vulva can never measure up to a picture of one. Thank you to everyone who filled this book with images: Christopher M. Brown, Catherine Johnson-Roehr, Rachel Liebert, Melissa Nannen, and Maleese N. Schick.

We feel fortunate to be surrounded by colleagues who inspire us daily. In particular, we would like to thank Michael Reece, Brian Dodge, and everyone at the Center for Sexual Health Promotion for their enthusiasm, their willingness to listen to and give feedback on our ideas, and the way they embrace our vulva puppets and other unique office decor. We would like to thank David Lohrmann and Mohammad Torabi, who have established an academic work environment in which our research and creative interests are able to thrive. We are also appreciative of the support we have received from Jenny Bass, Dennis Fortenberry, Carol McCord, Heather Rupp, Stephanie Sanders, and Shawn Wilson, among others. We would be remiss not to thank Chelsea Heaven for her careful, conscientious work.

This book would not have been possible without the many women and men who have inspired us at different points in our personal and professional development. Although not limited to the following, we like to acknowledge the work and vision of (in alphabetical order) Joani Blank, Virginia Braun, Judy Chicago, Betty Dodson, Eve Ensler, Nick and Sayaka Karras, Dorrie Lane, Rachel Liebert, Carol Queen, Wrenna Robertson, Carlin Ross, Annie Sprinkle, Elizabeth Stewart, Leonore Tiefer, and Chris Veasley.

We would like to express our heartfelt gratitude to everyone who took the time to share personal stories about their thoughts, feelings, and experiences with vulvas and vaginas, whether for *Read My Lips* or for the various research projects we have conducted over the years.

Vanessa would like to thank everyone who has supported or inspired her along this spectacular journey. First, she would like to thank her phenomenal co-author, Debby Herbenick, who made this possible. There is only enough light for everyone to share if you open your door and let others in. She is forever grateful for Debby's encouragement, guidance, humor, and perpetual kindness. She would also like to thank her graduate advisor, Alyssa Zucker, who encouraged her to follow her passion; Laina Bay-Cheng, who continuously challenged her to think about things in new and complex ways; and Maria-Cecilia Zea, who urged her to see the potential in herself. On a personal note, Vanessa would like to thank her friends and family for all of their support, love, and friendship throughout this process. She is particularly grateful to the following: Ashley, Bindi, Geneva, Heather, Jenn, Kelly, and Marcela for their constant friendship, encouragement, and quick feedback on the cover. Vanessa would also like to thank Sarah, for being the amazing person she is both professionally and personally. She makes quirky seem normal. Russell/Thaddeus, for always being patient, proud, and the biggest bighead she has ever known. M. T. McGillicutty, for (sometimes) holding it during long writing sessions and cuddling even when she didn't want to. Her many brothers and sisters, who inspire her in ways they can only imagine. Her aunt Bobbie, who always says the right thing at the right moment. Her belated grandmother and step-mother, for always being outspoken and strong. Her father, for encouraging her to work hard at what she believed in. Her mother, for believing in her and inspiring Vanessa to make her journey her own.

Debby would like to thank the following individuals for their particular support of her vulva and vagina outreach: Vanessa Schick, for bringing her talent, brilliance, and spunk to Indiana University, and for being an amazing co-author on this book; Stephanie Sanders, for being the first mentor to support her interest in vulvovaginal research; June Reinisch, for pointing her in the direction of positive vulva references in historical texts and for her enthusiastic mentorship; the late Joe Miller, for his support of her initial research about attitudes toward women's genitals; Tyra Banks, for inviting Debby to share her vulva puppet and vulvovaginal information with her television audience; Kareen Gunning, for her commitment to educating the masses about women's health and sexual health; Patty Brisben, for her passionate support of research and education related to women's sexual health; Dan Savage, for enduring assorted vulva-related conversations and puppetry; and Annie, Debbie, Joyce, Mary, and Paulene, for their steadfast support, dependability, and good natures. In addition, Debby would like to express her enormous gratitude to her mother and sister for their consistent support during the past decade-plus of her vagina/vulva outreach journey. She would like to acknowledge the memory of her maternal grandmother who encouraged her in the study of women's sexual health and vulvovaginal perceptions, and her father who was one of her biggest sources of support in all areas of life. She is grateful to Jezebel, who stayed up late with her while writing, to those who have helped her to love her vulva and vagina (including the dozens of women, such as Jada, Sarah, and Jessica, with whom she worked on *The Vagina Monologues*), and her gynecologist, who has helped her to care for it. Finally, Debby would like to thank Ariane, Brooke, Brandon, Rachel, Kate, Tom, Ben, Susie, Erica, Roberta, and Jimmy, all of whom have shown their support by listening to vulva/vagina stories, helping to select cover designs, or making space for her to write this book. No one, however, has listened to as many vulva stories or made as much space for this work (or for vulva craft projects) as James, for whom she is eternally grateful.

With much vulva love to you all,
Debby & Vanessa

Introduction

$\mathcal{I}$t was a warm November evening as the sun set in San Juan, Puerto Rico. The ocean crashed in the background as a light breeze swept through the air. If this sounds like the makings of a magical night, it was indeed: this is the night that we (Debby and Vanessa) first met. But this isn't a love story—at least, not the kind you might expect.

We were both in San Juan, Puerto Rico, attending the annual meeting of the Society for the Scientific Study of Sexuality. Although the field of sexuality researchers is small, the number of people who study social and cultural issues related to vaginas and vulvas is even smaller and was almost non-existent several years ago. Therefore, we assumed that like other conferences, we would probably be the only vulva researchers there. We were wrong. We had been at the conference for just minutes when a colleague who was familiar with both of our work introduced us. It took just one phrase to bond us instantaneously, and it went something like this: "You two should meet—you both study vaginas."

So yes, this is a love story about vulvas and vaginas.

Once we met, it wasn't long before we realized how much we had in common: we had both conducted our dissertation research on women's genitals, and we both have stuffed vulva puppets and books with titles like *Cunt* and *The V Book* lining our office bookshelves. With these mutual interests, it was only a matter of time—less than a year—before we found a way to work together, thanks to Vanessa taking a position at the Center for Sexual Health Promotion at Indiana University, where Debby had been working for several years. Shortly thereafter, the idea for *Read My Lips* was born, and after much work, brainstorming over lunches, and 2 a.m. email exchanges, it's now in your hands.

This book is for anyone who has a vulva, loves someone with a vulva, has come from a vagina, or is just plain curious about these parts. Through our research and education efforts, we try to better understand the diverse ways in which women's genitals are talked about (or not), and we try to help women and men learn about this important part of the female body in terms of health, sex, pleasure, culture, and art. In addition to working as scientific researchers, we also feel passionately about spreading the word to others, which is why we decided to write a book to share with the world. We like to refer to this as vagina and vulva "outreach."

What does this mean for you? It means that your journey will be filled with the unusual combination of empirical scientific research, quirky humor, and vulva crafts. In addition to assembling some of the most interesting scientific research we could find, we also turned to more than one thousand other experts on the topic of vulvas and vaginas: YOU! These pages are filled with funny, heartwarming, eye-opening, and sometimes challenging stories from women and men who live all over the world, ages eighteen to eighty. We chose stories that we felt best represent the complexity of what it means to live life with these body parts: to take in what parents and friends say to young girls about their bodies, to witness how lovers respond to vulvas and vaginas, and to experience the ways in which these parts change during menstruation, after giving birth, or as one ages.

We should note that even though women, vulvas, and vaginas almost always go together, this isn't always the case. Some women don't have vulvas or vaginas from the time they were formed in the womb (they may have what are sometimes called a disorder of sex development or intersex condition) or because they are male-to-female transgendered people who may identify as women but who have not had surgery to change their genitals to female-typical genitals. For similar reasons related to development or gender identity, some people who have vulvas and vaginas are men, not women. Although we tried to be sensitive to these issues in our book, we often use the phrases "women's genitals" and "female genitals" to refer to vulvas and vaginas even though these are not always interchangeable. We did this for two reasons: (1) most of the time they are interchangeable, and so this will make sense to most readers of our book; and (2) to avoid overkill, we varied the terms we used. This is also why we sometimes use genital slang such as "coochie," "twat," "snatch," "v-parts," "down there," "private parts," "lady parts," and other such words. Just because we know the technical terms for the vulva and vagina doesn't mean that we always want to use them. Sometimes we like using fun words, too, just like the one-thousand-plus women and men who completed our survey and told us about the many words that they use for vulvas and vaginas.

We wrote *Read My Lips* because we wanted to write the kind of book that we wish we had come across earlier in our lives. It has a little bit of everything, including information about the parts of the vulva, health issues, sex, pubic hairstyles, periods, smell, taste, appearance, GYN exams, genital self-image, orgasms, feminine-hygiene products, and art. It also uses crafting, a traditionally female form of expression, to engage in the somewhat subversive act of celebrating and exploring issues related to the often contested territory of vulvas and vaginas.

We hope that you will enjoy and embrace our labor of v-love for what it is: a celebration of and an education about the vulva and vagina. We hope that you laugh while you read this book and also that you walk away from each chapter feeling as though you've learned something new. We hope, too, that your reading inspires you to love and respect your vulva and vagina (or those of a partner or friend) as the beautiful, powerful, and sometimes magical places that they can be.

Meet the Vulva

$\mathcal{L}$ike love, the vulva is a many-splendored thing. In addition to quite literally serving as the window to a baby's world during vaginal birth, women's genitals are also often a source of pleasure, stimulation, and orgasmic release. Although women who look at, touch, and appreciate their vulvas and vaginas may be particularly well situated to experience genital pleasure, women who have never seen or touched their genitals can start exploring at any time (well, almost any time; it's wise and considerate of others to wait until you're alone or with a partner rather than try this at work, on public transportation, or at the grocery store).

That said, vulvas have a complicated history. There are reasons why some women may feel uncomfortable or unfamiliar with this part of their own bodies. Although some people in certain cultures have done or continue to do harmful things to women's genitals, the vulva has long been revered, adored, and even worshipped by many people and in many societies.[1, 2] We're here to tell you why, how, and in what interesting ways this has been done, including a story about the time we took to the famous Las Vegas Strip with Vanessa dressed in a self-made and way larger-than-life vulva costume while Debby conducted on-camera interviews with adult women and men of all ages about vulvas.[3]

V-CRAFT: DIY VULVA COSTUME

In September 2009, when Vanessa and Debby walked up and down the Las Vegas Strip with Vanessa dressed as a giant vulva,[3] we got so many great reactions to our experiment (check out our video podcasts on our web site—readmylipsthebook.tumblr.com—to see how people responded to us). We didn't know what would happen: Would people look at us funny? Would they laugh? Would we get arrested for a public vulva display? We truly had no idea.

Although a few people thought Vanessa was dressed as a *Star Wars* character, many people knew exactly what she was—and they were thrilled. One man, a professional poker player from Japan—said that she was dressed as "the best thing in the world," which warmed our hearts.

Here's how to create your own vulva costume:

What You'll Need

- two pairs of tights (can be any color)
- four sheets (can be from the same set or different sets)
- some scissors
- a vulvariffic attitude

Vulva newbies will probably want to read this book two or three times, as their new knowledge about women's genitals soaks in. However, even the most seasoned, well-versed vulvalucionaries will find new facts about women's genitals in these pages as they're informed by the latest and greatest recent discoveries about women's vulvas and vaginas. And who doesn't need a new vulva craft project? (You'll find at least one craft project nestled in each chapter.) First, though, let's get acquainted with the vulva so that we can begin our adventure together with a shared sense of knowledge.

What to Do

1. Stuff the sheets into the legs of the two pairs of tights. One sheet goes in each leg.
2. Knead the sheet-filled tights to bunch the labia any way you like. Remember: labia can be any shape or size, and they are rarely ever symmetrical.
3. If you would like to bring your hair through the tights (so as to resemble pubic hair once it is on), use scissors to cut one or more small holes in the crotch of the pantyhose. Cut the hole before the tights are on your head, or you run the risk of accidentally cutting yourself. Always be careful when holding scissors near real or fake genitals!
4. Slip the crotch area of the tights over your head—almost so that it looks like a bald wig—and slip your hair through the holes, if desired.
5. Once both pairs are on over your head, tie the toes of the tights down around your waist or wherever they fall so that the labia stay together.
6. Your head is the clitoris, so smile and be proud!

For more specifics, check out our DIY Vulva Costume video on our web site.

WHAT'S A VULVA?

If you guessed a car, we understand why; this is a common misperception given how close "vulva" and "Volvo" sound. However, the term "vulva" actually refers to the parts of a woman's genitals that can be seen from the outside: the mons pubis, clitoral hood, clitoris, labia majora, labia minora, and the introitus, also called the vaginal opening (the gateway to the vagina). If you're not sure what all these parts are or what they do, don't worry—you'll soon find out. Many women lack familiarity with their vulva parts. We certainly didn't always know a lot about vulvas, but we're happy that we learned about them so that we can spread the word to other women and men. Case in point: years ago, when Debby was a graduate student at Indiana University (IU), she was tossing a Frisbee with her teammates from the Calamity Janes (IU's ultimate Frisbee club team) and talking about her sex-education work and what it was like to teach human sexuality classes to college students when one of her teammates asked her where the clitoris is located. Because Debby was standing in the middle of a grassy field without a textbook, diagram, or chalkboard in sight to use as a visual aid, she was forced to improvise.

People should learn what the vulva is. In the common mind, the vulva is called vagina. I spoke about this to an educated woman who was confused about the distinction between vulva and vagina. I had to get out an anatomy book to convince her. In another incident I had occasion to talk to a sex therapist. She admitted being guilty of referring to the vulva as vagina. The word vagina is now used freely. I heard Robin Williams on a TV show refer to 'vagina' meaning vulva. I must say, this makes me angry. It is denial in the guise of freedom to discuss sexuality in public.

—Joy, 82, New York

"Imagine my face is a vulva," Debby said, dropping the Frisbee to the ground. Pointing to her mouth, she said, "My mouth would be the vagina and my lips would be the labia minora, which are the inner vaginal lips." Next, she pushed her cheeks closer to her lips and said, "My cheeks would be the labia majora, the outer vaginal lips. That would make my nose—just above the vagina but not inside of it—my clitoris."

Not only did Debby's Frisbee teammates learn about the vulva and clitoris that day, but Debby also invented a new way to use her face as an educational icebreaker at parties and a great get-to-know-each-other topic on first dates. Try it sometime (well—maybe not on "first" dates).

Watch a video of Debby showing how her face can become a vulva on our web site, www.readmylipsthebook.tumblr.com

Fortunately, we have diagrams available to us here in this book, so there's no need to rely on Debby's face for our entire knowledge about women's vulvas. Check out our diagrams to see where the various vulva parts are located. Then, if you're a woman, find some time to check out your own vulva (if you're a man with a female sex partner, perhaps she will be kind enough to give you a guided tour of her vulva). In San Francisco, at the Center for Sexuality and Culture, gay men (mostly—but others are invited) have been able to sign up for and attend a class called "Cunts for Fags."[4] This class teaches attendees everything they need to know about vulvas and vaginas so that they can effectively teach about women's genitals alongside a

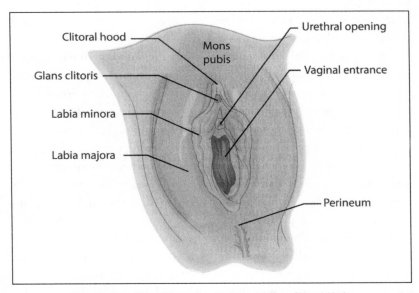

Diagram of the Vulva (Christopher M. Brown, Office of Visual Media, Indiana University School of Medicine)

wide range of sexual health topics. Those who have never previously seen a woman's vulva or vagina before are invited to view and/or touch genitals for educational purposes. If you are interested in attending, find more information from the Center for Sex and Culture (see Resources). We highly recommend the class for everyone regardless of whether you choose to have sex with a vulva-equipped woman.

As you review the diagrams, notice that, if you're a woman, your genital parts probably look a little or a lot different than the images here in this book. This is to be expected. After all, there is no one "standard" vulva[5–8]—a message that is worth repeating. Let's try that: *There is no one "standard" vulva.* This is a powerful message. It means that there is no need to compare the appearance of your genitals to the genitals of any other woman on the planet. Like a thumbprint, they are all a little different. Some women have a small glans clitoris (the part of the clitoris that can be seen from the outside), while other women have a glans clitoris that stretches out for an inch or two or more. Most of us are somewhere in between. The size, color, and shape of the clitoral hood can vary, too.[5–8]

Only a handful of researchers have measured women's genital parts, but those that have done so have found that vulva parts come in all sorts of shapes and sizes (see sidebar). The labia minora (inner vaginal lips) are particularly variable in size.[8] Author, sex educator, and activist Betty Dodson used the name of famous architectural designs (e.g., baroque, classical) to emphasize the different, yet beautiful, variations in women's inner labia.[9] She, along with other sex educators and artists, has also likened the shape of women's labia to the appearance of hearts, angel wings, sea shells, or flowers (particularly orchids). Before we get too excited about the labia, though (and believe us, we definitely get going talking about labia in chapter 4), let's back up and go part by part through the vulva. Even if you think you know all your vulva parts, read on, as you may learn something new. Research scientists are learning new things about vulvas and vaginas all the time. Has there ever been a better time in the history of the world to have, or be curious about, a vulva?

VULVA DIMENSIONS

Several years ago, researchers measured the vulvas of fifty premenopausal women in order to better understand how similar and different
we all are from one another.[8] Here are some examples of what they
found in terms of female genital diversity.

Let's start with the clitoris:

- The length of the glans clitoris ranged from 3 to 35 mm.
- The width of the glans clitoris ranged from 3 to 10 mm.
- The distance from the clitoris to the urethra was as little as 14
  mm and as much as 45 mm.

Women's labia also varied considerably:

- The outer labia (labia majora) length ranged from 7 to 12 mm.
- Women's inner labia (labia minora) length ranged from 20 to
  100 mm.
- The width of the inner labia was as little as 7 and as much as 50 mm.

The size of the perineum ranged in length from 15 to 55 mm. The
researchers also noted the color of the genital area and how dark or
light it was compared with the color of women's surrounding skin. Of
the fifty women they examined, they found that nine women (18 percent) had genital skin that was the same color of the rest of their surrounding skin and forty-one had genital skin that was darker than the
skin around it.

VULVA INTRODUCTIONS

The **mons pubis** (a.k.a. "the mons") is a term that refers to the
triangular area between a woman's legs and is the genital part that
women have most frequently seen on other women, such as while
changing in the locker room. Other terms for this area include the
mound of Venus and the *pubic mound*. Most women, if they let nature
take its course, will have pubic hair growing on their mons and

down the outer edges of their **labia majora**, which are women's outer vaginal lips, as well as a little or a lot of pubic hair on the inner thighs.[10] For women who choose to keep some or all of their pubic hair, it can feel sensuous to gently tug on one's pubic hair during masturbation or sex with a partner.

WHAT'S IN A NAME?

Debby used to prefer the term "labia minora" to describe a woman's inner vaginal lips. After all, labia minora was the correct clinical term so it must be better, right? That's what Debby thought, anyway. Then she met Vanessa and the world as she knew it changed.

Vanessa had previously been at a conference talking about her labia research when a person pointed out how problematic the language was that she was using. Instead, he suggested that perhaps we should all use "inner labia" and "outer labia" rather than "labia minora" and "labia majora." Why?

Well, labia can vary in size. And although the inner lips are sometimes smaller than (and thus "minor" as compared to) the outer lips (the labia majora), this is not always the case. This man, and then Vanessa, felt we could be setting women up for misperceptions about their bodies if the term "labia minora" suggests that inner lips should be small.

After thinking about it in this way, Debby and Vanessa have both tried to use the terms "inner labia" or "inner lips" more often when referring to the labia minora, though old habits can die hard. If you see us out and about and using the term "labia minora," give us a nudge in the right direction, will you?

The outer labia encase the inner parts of the vulva, such as the clitoris, clitoral hood, and the vaginal entrance. However, there is some variability in terms of the size, shape, and color of women's outer and inner labia.[8] The **labia minora**, which are also sometimes called the inner vaginal lips, are sometimes smaller than the labia majora (or outer vaginal lips) and sometimes longer than the labia majora.

Not a lot of women and men know this because, as Vanessa discovered in a research study that she and her colleagues at George Washington University in Washington, DC, conducted, inner labia that hang down lower than the outer labia are often missing from sexually explicit magazines such as *Playboy*—probably thanks to digital editing or airbrushing techniques.[11] If the famous fictional detective Nancy Drew were more progressive and took on vulva-related cases, there would perhaps be a story called *The Case of the Missing Labia*.

As a result of inner labia that are mostly missing or airbrushed out of porn and other sexual images, many people don't know how creative nature has been with women's genitals and what a wide range of labia exist in the wild—and by "the wild" we mean in women's bedrooms, apartments, tents, and mud huts around the world. Vulvas are incredibly diverse—just like faces. No wonder so many artists have portrayed women's genitals with such beauty and reverence.[6, 12]

VULVARIATIONS

The inner labia (labia minora) are perhaps the most diverse part of women's genitals. The color of women's inner labia may vary greatly from one woman to the next.[8] They may be a shade of pink, red, brown, gray, black, or slightly purple (particularly as women become sexually aroused and blood flow increases to the genitals, as the inner labia are filled with blood vessels; inner labia also sometimes darken in color while a woman is pregnant). The outer ridges of the inner labia are often darker than the rest of the labia. Similarly, in one study, forty-one of fifty women (92 percent) had genitals that were darker than the skin around their genitals.[8]

Like a woman's eyes, ears, and breasts, women's inner labia are usually not symmetrical. One labium (the singular version of labia) may be longer, differently shaped, or differently "textured" compared to the other one. It is critical to understand that this is a normal part of development. Because the inner labia don't have fat in them (unlike with outer labia, which contain fat that acts like padding to keep the genitals safe and comfortable), the inner labia are thinner and may lay in ways that give them the appearance of assorted shapes. In fact, the inner labia can take on a variety of shapes depending on how one holds them up or down or to the sides. If you have a full-length mirror, you might find it interesting to sit in front of it (make sure the room is well lit), spread your legs open enough so that you can view your genitals, and then see how the way you touch or hold your labia can make them look symmetrical one way, asymmetrical another way, like a heart or flower, or as if your vulva has angel wings.

I wish there was more information on how women's genitals actually look. All you see in a health class is STD-infected genitals and it is gross to look at them. I would have liked to [have seen] some pictures of healthy genitals and maybe some starting not so close up (with a partner perhaps) and then closer up to ease you in. They also NEVER show you a picture of how genitals look when they are together (sex), because they consider that porn. I would have loved to see how genitals move and stretch when people are having sex and how the vulva looks different in various sexual activities (masturbation, oral sex, vaginal sex).
—KELLY, 28, New York

Some women worry that something is wrong with them if one labium is bigger than the other one, but we're here to tell you that that's not the case. "Even if nothing's wrong," some women have said to us, "I still wish they were the same size." Fair enough. But consider for a moment that some people look for each other's quirks, eccentricities, or special unique aspects of appearance to love. You might think of a past or current lover whose freckles form a constellation or come together to look like a paw print and how that special way you re-imagined your partner's body made you glow with love or attraction. If you feel self-conscious about your genitals, try to imagine how someone else might look upon them with love or adoration. What you view as quirky or unusual, another person may view as special and unique. For example, a friend of ours once mentioned that his wife told him that she felt self-conscious about the dark edges of her inner labia. She had considered surgery to get rid of the darker edges. This surprised our friend because he had always thought that the dark edges of her inner labia were particularly sexy and appealing. Until they talked about this, he didn't know that she didn't like her inner labia, and she didn't know that he thought they were beautiful just as they are. (This is also an example of how communicating with one's partner about his or her body and about sexuality can help a couple's sex life and relationship.) A woman we know had a boyfriend who had a birthmark on his penis, which he felt self-conscious about. However, she couldn't imagine his penis any other way and loved that he had this special, unique part of his body that she knew about but the rest of the world did not; it made her feel special.

People have all sorts of individual aspects to their genitals. Some people—like the man we just told you about—have a birthmark (an area of darker pigmented skin) on their genitals. Many men find that their penis, when erect, bends upward or downward or to the side. Like vulva variations, the degree and direction of "bend" can be a normal and common difference among men and is nothing that needs to cause feelings of embarrassment or shame.[13]

I just remembered that I have a freckle just outside my labia. I really like it.
—KARA, 20, Tonga

Many women, if they look closely at their inner labia, might notice that their left labium is larger or longer than their right—a trait that is common to many men, too, who often find that their left testes hang lower than their right. For some women, it may be the right labium that is larger or that hangs down lower than the left. People are diverse!

When Your Labia Hurt

There are times when women may have inner labia that cause them discomfort or pain. In rare instances, a woman may find that the length or thickness of her inner labia gets in the way of masturbation or vaginal intercourse, or that her inner labia get uncomfortably pushed up inside the vagina during vaginal penetration.[14] Although some women wonder if surgery to make the labia smaller will help, this is not always the case. Even women with very tiny inner labia— smaller than one centimeter of length—can experience this "pushing inside" effect during sex.

Surgery is not always an effective solution for labia that are pushed inside during sex (and any surgery carries costs and risks of surgical or other health complications). As such, it may be effective for women and their partners to take their time to gently begin penetration. Once penetration begins (whether a woman is having vaginal intercourse or enjoying finger or sex-toy penetration with a partner) and care has been taken to penetrate in a way that doesn't cause discomfort or push the inner labia uncomfortably inside the vagina, sexual play may be more comfortable. Then—and only then—both partners may be ready to go faster, switch from gentle to rougher sex, or explore their sexuality in some other way they find pleasurable. If the inner labia get pushed inside the vagina, a woman and her partner can briefly stop sex to readjust. People take sex "breaks" all the time for many different reasons, and it needn't disrupt sex or feel awkward. When you take a sex break, you always have the opportunity to switch positions, apply or reapply lubricant, get a sip of water, or use the towel trick (more on the towel trick later).

In other rare instances, some women may find that their inner labia cause significant discomfort, chafing, or pain during everyday activities such as walking long distances, running, or wearing tight clothing.[14–16] As a last resort for women with pain, some doctors offer a surgical procedure called a labiaplasty—essentially, a reshaping and resizing of the inner labia—to women as a means of improving their situation. Not all doctors have significant experience performing labiaplasty. If you are interested in learning more about this procedure, we recommend that you contact our favorite vulvovaginal society—the International Society for the Study of Vulvovaginal Disease (www.ISSVD.org; 704.814.9493)—to find a doctor who is an expert in vulvovaginal health. Women may also choose to have a labiaplasty for aesthetic reasons, such as to remove darkened edges or make their labia more symmetric (social critiques of the surgery are discussed in chapter 4). However, many healthcare providers believe that this decision should be made with extreme care and after consulting with a doctor who has expertise in vulvovaginal health. After all, every surgery carries risks, and surgery to the genitals is certainly no exception.[17] As more doctors advertise labiaplasty (and thus more women appear to be asking for the procedure), scientists are just now catching up in terms of conducting research about the surgery, such as the potential risks, benefits, and outcomes. One doctor even went so far to compare the field of female elective genital surgery to the "old Wild, Wild West" because it is currently "wide open and unregulated."[18] Once again, we recommend connecting with a member of the ISSVD for additional information.

THE CLITORIS: IS IT REALLY THAT COMPLEX?

When we teach about the vulva, most people want to zero right in on the clitoris (kind of like during sex play with a new partner who fumbles around down there). People are often very interested in learning about the clitoris given the glitz and glamour of the world it inhabits. What's that, you say? The clitoris lives in a world of glitz and glamour? In some ways, it does. Unlike many Hollywood celebrities, the clitoris gets a ton of press without even trying: it's mentioned almost monthly in popular women's and men's magazines, and it doesn't even have a publicist or a drug problem. So, why all the hoopla?

The clitoris gets a lot of play because, frankly, it seems built for play, as we'll talk about more in later chapters. The clitoris also gets significant media attention because scientists are constantly learning new things about this very important part of women's bodies. The sole function of the clitoris is to serve as a place of sensation, pleasure, and orgasm. It has nothing to do with urination, menstruation (periods), or the birthing process. It only serves a "feel good" function (packed with about eight thousand nerve endings).

I wish that they didn't seem so foreign. I know what's what down there and the general idea of how they work, but at the same time they're so confusing. I think understanding the mechanics of things would help a lot. Just like how you know how your hands work, how hands should work and what the normal differences between them are, it would be nice to be able to feel that comfortable with genitals.

—SUSIE, 18, Illinois

Scientists continue to study the clitoris because there seem to be more questions about it than answers. Although people used to only think of the clitoris in terms of the part one can see from the outside of the body (that little one-quarter to one-half-inch nubbin), the clitoris is much larger than that—something that became more widely

---

YOU SAY VULVA, I SAY VAJAYJAY

People have all sorts of words that they use to describe women's genitals or specific genital parts, such as the clitoris or labia. When we've taught college students, we've sometimes asked them to list all the slang terms that they know for both women's and men's genitals. Then, we discuss the terms as a class. This can be a particularly valuable exercise in a mixed-gender class, as it may be the first time that some students have heard women voice their feelings of discomfort or offense with terms for women's genitals that are violent (e.g., "ax wound") or passive (e.g., "receptacle").[19] It also provides a space for women to talk about the words that help them to feel that their genitals are places of pleasure and beauty that they should feel proud about. In addition, students get a chance to talk about their divergent views on certain terms, such as "cunt" or "pussy," that are loved by some and hated by others.

One of our favorite terms for women's genitals has long been "Little Miss Sassy"—one that we first heard in a research study that Debby conducted years ago at The Kinsey Institute. If you're curious about female-genital slang, you may find it interesting to read through

known in 1998 when an Australian researcher named Helen O'Connell published a scientific paper that illustrated the full size of the clitoris.[20] Inside a woman's body, there are various parts of the clitoris that work together to enlarge during sexual arousal and to somehow function as part of the female orgasm process (a process that remains pretty mysterious).

More recently, Dr. O'Connell has suggested that perhaps a new name be used to describe the clitoris and the surrounding bodies: the name she suggests is "the clitoral complex."[21] This is because the vagina, urethra, and clitoris appear to move hand-in-hand (or "clit-urethra-vag"?). Essentially, it seems that one cannot move or stimulate one of these three parts without moving or stimulating the other parts. This means that when a woman experiences penile-

---

some of the terms we've heard in our classes and also in our research. For better or worse, the terms include:

pink taco	cunt	little girl	bits
vajayjay	twat	V-parts	lady bits
cooch	little man in a boat	down there	gina
poonanny	muffin	downstairs	coochie hole
front bum	warm penis holder	hooha	minge
fanny	waa-waa	Little Miss Sassy	receptacle
snatch	man eater	honeypot	button
kitten	ditty	pussy	slit
vertical smile	vagotch	clam	flower
cockpit	fluffy taco	poontang	box
special place	pleasure zone	lower lips	cooter
innie penis	privates	beaver	sideways smile
lady garden	choche	fish taco	ax wound
yoni	poomps	mitt	bush
passarinha	womanhood	pipi	muschi
sexy	"you know"	love button	bald spot
girlie parts	stuff	wetness	pubic area
my sweet vulva	kitty cat	the V	smoothie
pleasure dome			

vaginal intercourse, her male partner's penis is not only stimulating her vagina but is moving inside her in a way that also moves her urethra and clitoris (even if the penis does not touch these parts directly). This may also explain, at least in part, why some women feel as though they have to urinate when they are in the midst of intercourse or approaching orgasm. The penis may be indirectly stimulating the urethra (and maybe the bladder, too), as well as the nerves in these areas. For a more detailed discussion of orgasm and the nerve pathways, we recommend reading *The Science of Orgasm.*[22]

THE VAG IN ALL

Although the vaginal entrance is often technically called the "introitus" in medical circles, another name for it and the area just around it is the "vestibule"—coincidentally, this is also the name for the entrance to a church. In fact, some people have likened churches to vulvas in their design and in their ability to give birth to new life.

The Hymen

The vaginal opening of most girls' bodies is partially covered with a thin layer of tissue called the hymen, which—although thin—is filled with blood vessels. It is important to note that the hymen does not fully cover the vaginal opening. If it did, a girl's vagina would not be able to easily self-clean through the release of vaginal discharge. When a healthcare provider notices that a girl's hymen completely covers her vaginal opening, he or she may wait to see if it resolves later during childhood or around the time of puberty. If it does not, a healthcare provider will often perform a procedure to create an opening so that when a woman menstruates, the blood and tissue have a way to leave the body. Otherwise, the blood can back up and create feelings of pain and pressure in a woman's abdominal or pelvic area.

Some girls are not born with a hymen or are born with only a small amount of hymen tissue. Even girls who are born with a hymen may find that it wears away or tears during non-sexual activities during childhood or adolescence. A young woman may, without realizing it, tear her hymen while using tampons or during vaginal fingering that occurs as part of masturbation or sex play with a partner. As such, not all women notice vaginal bleeding when they first experience vaginal penetration or intercourse. Unfortunately, some people mistakenly believe that if a woman does not bleed when she first has intercourse that she must not truly have been a virgin. This is problematic for many reasons including those related to sexual double standards that suggest that women should be virgins until they get married but that men don't have to be virgins at the time of marriage. Also, women in some cultures are pressured to "prove" their virginity, whereas men typically are not pressured to "prove" theirs, probably because there is no way to "prove" their virginity by looking at their penis or scrotum. If only more people realized that there is no sure way to "prove" women's virginity either!

Even women who are not waiting to have sex until they are married sometimes feel confused if they have intercourse and don't notice any blood. We have heard from women who wonder what it means when they don't bleed the first time they have sex. They may ask, for example, if they are still virgins if they have had sex but didn't bleed from it. Or they may ask if something is physically wrong with them if they did not bleed when they first had intercourse. A lack of bleeding at first sex does not necessarily mean that there is anything wrong with a woman or her body; vulvas and vaginas vary, just as women do, and not all women bleed when they first have sex, particularly if the hymen has been worn away from other activities.

Recently, in some countries, a procedure called a hymenoplasty has increased in popularity. It involves surgically placing new tissue over part of a woman's vaginal opening as if it were a hymen. A woman might choose to have this procedure in an effort to try and "prove" to her new husband or his family that she is a virgin, even though she has previously (and perhaps secretly) had vaginal intercourse. Other women who are sexually experienced choose to have a hymenoplasty so that they can feel as though they are re-experiencing their virginity loss with a new partner. We know of a woman who chose to have this procedure done as an anniversary present for her husband, as neither one of them had been virgins when they met or married, and she wanted to experience the feeling of him taking her "virginity" (to her, this meant that she wanted to experience him penetrating her by tearing her newly created "hymen"). Some people may be intrigued by this idea; others may feel that this is a lot of expense, recovery time, and possibly discomfort or pain to go through for an anniversary celebration. Others are concerned that the procedure perpetuates the sexual double standard that women should remain virgins. If the idea sounds like fun sexual play, but you'd rather not go through a surgical procedure and its accompanying costs, risks, and recovery time, why not consider placing a penetrable material (e.g., wax paper) over a pair of crotchless panties? Or engage in dirty-talk fantasy play in which you pretend you're involved in a devirginizing experience without actually breaking your hymen? A pain-free possibility!

The Vagina

The vagina is about three to four inches long when a woman is just hanging out and not feeling sexually aroused (it gets bigger during sexual arousal, but more on that later). At the far end of the vagina is the cervix, which is the opening to the uterus. The cervical opening is very small, which is why menstrual blood doesn't "gush" out of it the way that water flows out of a faucet.

I am teaching my daughters the proper terms for their bodies and the bodies of boys, with help from some terrific books with accurate illustrations. I also tell them that MOST girls have vulvas and MOST boys have penises, but not always. I want them to understand gender in complex ways. I tell them the [only] way to know someone's gender for certain is to ask.

—DEANNA, 41, Illinois

The vagina is not nearly as nerve-rich as the clitoris, which is probably a good thing as otherwise, vaginal birth might be a whole lot more painful than it already is for many women. Most of the nerve endings in the vagina are toward the vaginal entrance. Due to the lack of sensory nerve endings toward the back of the vagina, that part isn't very sensitive, which is why a woman can't generally feel a tampon or vaginal ring contraceptive (i.e., NuvaRing) inside her vagina if it's pushed back far enough.

Although the vagina has long-been described as a muscular "tube," research suggests that there may be several slightly different shapes for women's vaginas. It's not that there are dramatic differences between women's vaginas, with some being very large and others being quite small. Slight differences in shape may, in part, account for why some women enjoy certain sexual positions or types of vaginal stimulation and others do not. If you've ever had a friend who swears by a certain position that makes you go "meh," perhaps this helps explain some—but of course not all—of the differences between your experiences.

Fact!

The vagina, when unaroused, is only about three to four inches long.

What are these shapes, you ask? Well, there are five shapes identified thus far, and researchers have named them as follows: the heart, the pumpkin seed, the parallel sides, conical, and—get ready for this one—the slug. Why they ever thought that women would want their vagina to be named after a swamp creature, we'll never know, but there it is. (In November 2010, Debby talked about these shapes to

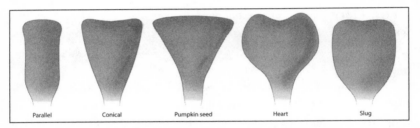

| Parallel | Conical | Pumpkin seed | Heart | Slug |

Five Shapes of Women's Vaginas (Christopher M. Brown, Office of Visual Media, Indiana University School of Medicine)

the cast of *The Doctors* on their television show, and they didn't seem too keen on the slug name either.)

Shapes aside, it's also true that these very same researchers didn't find dramatic differences between the vaginal sizes of different women. Women who had had babies didn't have vaginas that were any bigger overall than women who had not. So what accounts for differences in size and sensation if vaginas tend to be of a similar size? Several things might affect how vaginas feel, so read on!

LUBRICATION

Vaginal lubrication probably accounts for some of the differences in how "tight" or "loose" vaginas feel. After all, the wetter a woman's vagina is, the less friction there will be during sex, as natural vaginal lubrication does just that—it lubricates the vagina to decrease friction and thus decrease sensation. A vagina that is low on lubrication and is thus drier will be higher on friction and sensation, but this isn't always a good thing. According to our own research, women in the United States tend to prefer sex that feels pretty wet, as do most men, so there seems to be some happy medium that many women and their male or female partners strive for. Only you and your partner can determine what feels most pleasurable to you.

The Towel Trick

If vaginal intercourse or penetration with a sex toy feels pretty wet and as if there's not a whole lot of sensation, try dabbing a towel on both of your genitals (we call this the "towel trick"). By reducing some of the wetness, you may feel more "tight" and full of sensation. On the other hand, if your vagina feels too dry or as if sex is uncomfortable or full of too much unpleasant sensation, try spending more time during foreplay doing exciting things to promote vaginal lubrication. You can also add some personal lubricant (water-based or silicone-based may be preferable, especially if you are using condoms) in order to enhance wetness, comfort, and pleasure.

GENITAL FIT

For male-female couples, genital fit—how the penis and vagina fit together during intercourse—can also play a role in people's perceptions of vaginal size. A woman who has intercourse with a man who has a smaller-than-average-sized penis may feel as though sex (or her vagina) feels "roomy." However, that same woman could have sex with a man who has a larger-than-average-sized penis and wonder if her vagina is too small or too tight. Keep in mind: nothing about her vagina has changed. Neither the woman nor the men have "bad" genitals or genitals that are an undesirable size. Rather, the genital fit between partners can make sex feel different. So remember: there is no such thing as bad genital size, only a challenging genital fit. And even a challenging fit can be managed by adding lubricant, using the towel trick, or expanding one's ideas of sex to find other ways to experience fun, connection, and sexual pleasure. For example, a couple may experience greater pleasure through oral sex, sensual massage, the use of sex toys, or exploring sex positions that may help to make a tight genital fit more comfortable or a roomier genital fit feel more rich with sensation.

VAGINAL-WALL RELAXATION

Although many women say that six months or a year after giving birth, sex feels like it used to pre-pregnancy (except, of course, for the baby crying down the hall), other women have a different experience. Some women say that sex feels entirely different after they have been pregnant, whether or not they gave birth vaginally. Just being pregnant and bearing extra baby weight that's supported by one's pelvic-floor muscles may change the way that the vagina feels.

Unfortunately, some doctors have historically denied women's experiences in this regard and have told them things like "once you have a baby, nothing is ever the same again." Other providers may take matters into their own hands by providing the woman with a "husband stitch" during her episiotomy in order to "tighten" her vagina. Statements and actions like these can minimize women's feelings or make them feel as though they should put up with whatever uncomfortable or unpleasurable experiences they may be having, and we don't think that's right. We need a great deal more research to understand how women's bodies change after pregnancy and childbirth and what can be done to help them should they experience problems. We also need more healthcare providers trained to respond with sensitivity to women and with attention to how sex feels for them. Rather than dismissing a woman's experience by saying "nothing will ever be the same again" post-birth, we think it would be more helpful for that healthcare provider to ask follow-up questions, starting with, "Tell me how things are different for you now—what's changed?"

Research shows that with each additional birth, women are more likely to experience pelvic-floor distress symptoms, such as difficulties with incontinence. Often when women experience such pelvic-floor distress symptoms—a fancy term to describe a range of issues such as peeing when one doesn't mean to pee (incontinence), uncontrollably passing gas, or frequently needing to pee, among other symptoms—it is vaginal-wall relaxation that is at the root of the problem. The bladder may push through the front vaginal wall and create a slight bulge in it (the technical term is a "cystocele"). Or, the rectum may push against the back vaginal wall and create a slight bulge in the back wall (called a "rectocele"). Other terms you may hear used to describe these conditions are "prolapse" and "genital prolapse." Women who experience prolapse often report that sex lacks sensation. Some say that they can't feel their partner inside of them during sex. It's also the case that some women who experience prolapse, especially severe prolapse, avoid sex altogether because vaginal intercourse may increase their urge to pee or to have a bowel movement (which doesn't exactly make most women feel sexy).

Sometimes, women who undergo a surgical procedure commonly called a "front wall repair" or a "back wall repair" may notice an improvement across the board—both in terms of their pelvic-floor distress symptoms and their sensation during sex. If you've noticed a frequent or uncontrollable urge to pee or to have a bowel movement during sex or daily activities, or if you've noticed a significant decrease in sensation during sex, talk to your healthcare provider.

AROUSAL

A fourth factor that can affect how small or big a woman's vagina feels to her or her partner is how sexually aroused the woman herself feels—and how aroused she has allowed her body to become. Here's why arousal matters to the vagina:

When a woman is not sexually aroused or excited, her vagina is only about three to four inches long. For women who partner with men, and for women who engage in vaginal sex-toy play, this might not seem like much room. After all, most research on penis size suggests that the average erect penis is between five and six inches long.[23, 24] And sex toys such as dildos and insertive vibrators are often that length or longer. So, what gives?

Magic, that's what.

*I had my first girlfriend when I was fifteen; this was before I came out to my parents, and they didn't mind my having female friends over to stay the night. So she came over, and we went up to my room ("to watch a movie," supposedly), and locked the door. It was awkward, and embarrassing, and probably the most erotic experience I've ever had. I had touched her vulva before that, but that was the first time I'd actually **seen** it in good light.*

—AVA, 23, Vermont

When a woman becomes sexually aroused, her body begins to change. More blood flows to her genitals. Her heart rate and breathing increase. And her vagina? It lubricates and tents. Tents? Yes, tents. During sexual arousal, muscular tension pulls the uterus upward, which makes more room in a woman's vagina (after all, the uterus is at the far end of the vagina, so when it lifts up, more space is created). This process is called "vaginal tenting." It's a magical process because by making more space in the vagina, sex can feel more comfortable and pleasurable for many women who need a little more than three or four inches of space in order to accommodate their partner's penis or a favorite sex toy. This is one reason why spending more time in foreplay can help to make sexual intercourse with a penis or sex toy feel better. If a woman spends very little time in foreplay, her vagina might not have time to tent, and her vagina may feel unusually small, or the couple's genital fit may feel cramped for space. When a woman allows her body time to go through the process of vaginal tenting, there is the possibility that more space in the vagina will be created and that the couple's genital fit will be more comfortable.

HOW DO VAGINAS FEEL?

We can describe this all we want, but the only way to really get a sense is to feel your own vagina (if you have one) or to feel the vagina of a partner who is not only willing but who wants your finger or fingers in her vagina. You should never, of course, make someone feel bad for not wanting to do something sexual that you want to do.

So how do vaginas feel? Some might say "warm, wet, and a little bit bumpy." Vaginas—like some potato chips—have ridges in them, and yet, unlike potato chips, they tend to be warm and wet. Depending on a woman's age, the phase of her menstrual cycle (assuming she's still menstruating and has not yet reached menopause), and whether she is sexually aroused or not, a woman's vagina may feel slightly wet or very wet. Vaginal discharge may be clear and egg white-like in appearance, or it may be more thin and slick. Check it out and see what it feels like to you. In Debby's studies of men's and women's attitudes toward women's genitals (which is different than female genital self-image, described below), the majority of college students surveyed said that women's genitals felt good to touch.

VAGINA FACTS

There are a few more things you should know about the vagina in order to be well versed on the topic. For one, you should know that in addition to the way the vagina changes size during arousal, it can also change in structure with age. Specifically, the vagina typically rests at a 130-degree angle inside of pre-menopausal women's bodies. However, as women go through menopause, their bodies change and the vaginal angle flattens a bit, which may make vaginal intercourse feel different to women as they age and go through menopause.

Another important fact is that the vagina is a discreet space. The vagina starts at the vaginal opening and ends at the cervix, which is the opening to the uterus. The cervix has a very small opening in it, and there's not much other than fluids that can pass through it to go between the vagina and the uterus. Semen, of course, can pass through the cervix, as can menstrual fluids. And of course when a woman goes through labor to deliver a baby, then the baby can pass through the dilated cervix, but that is a very special circumstance. On a daily basis, the cervix is a small opening to the vagina, and the vagina remains a discreet space that's just three to four inches when unaroused and about two or three inches longer when aroused.

Why is this an important vagina fact to know? It means that objects such as condoms and diaphragms can't get "lost" inside the vagina. If a condom slips off a man's penis during sex and gets stuck in the vagina, then the woman or her partner can insert their fingers into her vagina to remove the condom. If they cannot find it, then the woman can ask a healthcare provider for help removing it (objects should always be removed from the vagina rather than left there as gravity will not draw them out on their own). By using her own fingers or getting help from her partner or healthcare provider, a woman should be able to retrieve anything else that she has put up there (though we don't recommend putting most foreign objects inside the vagina). This, of course, also goes for tampons (more in chapter 5) and Ben Wa balls, which some women use for sexual pleasure or as part of pelvic-floor exercises (more in chapter 2).

YOU LIKE, YOU LOVE?

Activity

Get out a piece of paper and a pen. Ready? Set? Okay, go—

Taking a stream-of-conscious approach to this activity, write down all the things that you like about your genitals. Think about smell, taste, sexy feelings, how you look. If you get stuck, write down some of the nice things that past or present partners have said about your genitals. Maybe they said that they liked how you smell or that you taste delicious. Maybe they liked how wet you get or how you squeezed their fingers or their penis with your pelvic-floor muscles. There are numerous reasons to appreciate one's own vulva and vagina, and all the parts within these parts (the clitoris, labia, etc.)—what are your reasons? What do you hope to change?

VAGINA CONTROVERSY

There are vagina facts, such as the fact that the vagina is about three to four inches long, and there are vagina myths, such as the myth that vaginas smell like fish (they don't, and we'll get to that later). Then there are vagina controversies. One of the biggest vagina controversies has to do with the G-spot. The G-spot was given its name in the 1980s, with the "G" referring to Dr. Grafenberg who, decades earlier in the 1950s, described an area on the front wall of the vagina that was full of erotic potential for some women. In 1982, the book *The G Spot: And Other Discoveries About Human Sexuality*[25] swept through the United States and many other countries with the message that sexual pleasure had to do with far more than the clitoral stimulation described by Kinsey[26] in the 1950s and Masters and Johnson[27] in the 1960s and 1970s. In *The G Spot*, readers discovered numerous stories of women who found stimulation of the front wall of the vagina to be particularly pleasurable and, for many, to be a reliable source of orgasm. For some, stimulation of this area—termed the G-spot—could also lead to the expulsion of fluids that came to be called female ejaculation.

So why the controversy? Isn't it a given that women vary in how they experience sex? After all, we're all different from each other.

The controversy lies in the fact that the G-spot is not a "thing" that can be seen. The G-spot is generally seen as something on the other side of the front vaginal wall—maybe it's the inside parts of the clitoris, or maybe it's the urethral sponge (tissue that surrounds the female urethra, just as spongy erectile tissue surrounds the male urethra in the penis). And when the front wall of the vagina is stimulated, often with firm but gentle pressure rather than a light flicking stimulation that the glans clitoris may respond to, the woman may feel wonderful things. In one study, 65 percent of women ages twenty-two to eighty-two in the United States and Canada felt that they had a particularly sensitive area in the vagina.

But if it can't be seen, then the G-spot is kind of like the Tooth Fairy to some people. Or to science-y folks, perhaps the G-spot is one big placebo effect that, if we believe it to be true, it becomes true and fun and possibly orgasm-inducing when stimulated.

One might think that with improvements in science the G-spot would become less controversial as more facts are gathered. However, that's not been the case. In 2008, Italian researchers using Magnetic Resonance Imaging (MRI) techniques, claimed they found that women who experienced orgasm from vaginal intercourse all by itself had a thicker urethrovaginal space (the area around the front wall of the vagina) than did women who do not experience orgasm from vaginal intercourse without extra stimulation, such as from a finger or sex toy.[28] In interviews, the researchers even suggested that perhaps MRI could be used as a "test" to find out if a woman had a G-spot or not. Some researchers (Debby included) felt that such statements were going well beyond the limited data they had collected from a very small study of only twenty women. And so this study largely became chalked up as interesting without necessarily telling us anything one way or the other about the G-spot.

Then in 2010, a team of researchers from the UK published a study suggesting that there is no G-spot—or at least no genetic basis for one, in spite of 56 percent of the women in their survey saying they had one.[29] They conducted a survey of 1,840 twin, heterosexual women in the UK, asking them, "Do you believe you have a so-called G-spot?" The fact that agreement among identical twins was no more common than among fraternal (non-identical) twins suggested to the researchers that there must be no physical basis to the G-spot. However, many researchers criticized this study, too. After all, a woman may believe or not believe in the existence of the "so-called G-spot" for any number of reasons including her own sexual experiences, things she has heard from friends or partners, human sexuality classes, or articles about the G-spot she has read in the media. Again, it was a curious study but it didn't close the gap in our understanding of the G-spot one way or the other.

To sum up, what we do know about the G-spot is this:

- It is clear that there is an area along the front wall of the vagina that some but not all women find to be pleasurable when stimulated with fingers, a penis, or a sex toy.
- There are undeniably body parts on the other side of the front vaginal wall (parts such as the internal parts (crura) of the clitoris, the urethral sponge, and their associated nerve endings) that may be stimulated through the front wall of the vagina.
- Large studies of women suggest that the majority of women feel they have a G-spot, or an area of erotic sensitivity on the front wall of the vagina.

As such, if you want to explore this area, go ahead! If you are a woman, you can try this on your own with your own fingers or with a sex toy. If you have a female partner, you might ask her if she would like to explore G-spot play, as well, with fingers, a sex toy, or

---

VIVA LA VULVA!

Activity

One of our favorite vulva-themed movies (and we have a few) is *Viva La Vulva*, created by vulva activist, educator, author, and artist Betty Dodson.[9] In *Viva La Vulva*, women come to Betty's home to be interviewed about their bodies, to groom (or not groom) their pubic hair in whatever way feels good to them, and to have their vulva portrait taken. One unique feature of this film is that the women—who span a few decades in age—go around and look at each other's vulvas, admiring them and remarking on various features such as the coloration of certain parts or the size or shape of the inner labia or clitoral hood. We have both shown this video in classes that we've taught, and male and female students alike often have a powerful reaction to watching even just twenty minutes of the film. We highly recommend you get a copy (see Resources).

(if you're a guy) with your penis. If it doesn't feel all that interesting or exciting to you, then perhaps move on to something else and try again (or not) another time. And if it does feel pleasurable to you, then yay for you! You've learned something new about your body that may enhance your sex life.

FEMALE EJACULATION

Another vagina controversy has to do with female ejaculation—and it doesn't even seem to be coming from the vagina (although for years, some wondered if female ejaculation came from the vagina, so we still consider it a "vagina controversy"). It seems that some women release fluids from their urethra during sexual excitement or orgasm. We don't know how common this experience is, as there have been no good population-based studies of women that would tell us with any certainty whether it's 10 percent of women, 40 percent of women, or nearly all women who are capable of female ejaculation.

Some people don't like the term "female ejaculation," as the fluids aren't exact matches for male ejaculation, and it is certainly a different process with different body parts involved. However, we use the term "female ejaculation" because it's commonly used in the United States and it's a term that many people are familiar with hearing described as such.

People vary in regard to how they feel about female ejaculation. Some people enjoy it and feel that female ejaculation is a huge turn-on. Others are uncomfortable with the amount of wetness it creates and may worry about getting their sheets wet (some people have similar concerns with male ejaculation). If you like the wetness, great! And if you're not a fan of it, you might want to lay a towel down on the bed before you masturbate or have sex. If it's a little unpredictable when you have sex, and you don't want to run to the towel closet on the spur of a moment, keep a few towels underneath your bed or in your nightstand for easy reach.

If you have never experienced female ejaculation, we don't recommend that you put any extra effort into trying—in spite of the popularity of some books and movies that try to show women how to go about doing this. Here's why: it's generally not a good idea to frequently bear down on your pelvic-floor muscles, as it may weaken them. Over time, everyone's pelvic-floor muscles weaken anyway, and this can lead to problems with incontinence (peeing when one doesn't mean to pee). Why hasten the process? Rather, if you feel that it is happening, let yourself go there if you want to try it. But we wouldn't recommend that you strain yourself—or your pelvic-floor muscles—trying to make it happen. There are enough pressures when it comes to sex; why add another one? Instead, try to focus on how your body works and enjoy your experience. People's sex lives changes over time, anyway, and you may end up experiencing female ejaculation one day without even trying. Stranger things have happened.

Finally, although chemical analyses of female ejaculate have shown that it is not the same as urine, some women can't help but wonder if they are peeing (by accident) during sex. If you have concerns about incontinence, for example, if you leak urine when you laugh or cough or if you feel as though you're often running to the bathroom through-out the day, check in with your healthcare provider. You might also try reducing or eliminating your caffeine intake, as caffeine can cause people to feel as if they frequently need to urinate (it does this by making the bladder muscle spasm).

PERINEUM

The perineum is the area between the bottom of a woman's vaginal entrance and her anus. It's also called the "taint" (as in, t'ain't the va-gina, t'ain't the anus) or the "tween" area (as it is "between" those two parts). In medical circles, you will hear it called the perineum. Most women won't ever hear people talking about their perineum. It's not a particularly sensitive or erotic spot for most women, although it is for some. More often, it comes into play because women who give birth vaginally may experience natural tearing of their perineum during childbirth or may have this area surgically cut during child-birth during a procedure called an "episiotomy." This procedure has become more controversial in recent years, and many women choose to talk to their healthcare providers and ask them not to perform an episiotomy unless absolutely necessary, as natural tears may heal better than surgical cuts. If you are pregnant, you may find it helpful to ask your healthcare provider or midwife about their take on episiotomies.

THE FEMALE GENITAL SELF-IMAGE SCALE (FGSIS)

The following items are about how you feel about your own genitals (the vulva and the vagina). The word "vulva" refers to a woman's external genitals (the parts that you can see from the outside such as the clitoris, pubic mound, and vaginal lips). The word "vagina" refers to the inside part, also sometimes called the "birth canal" (this is also the part where a penis may enter or where a tampon is inserted). Please indicate how strongly you agree or disagree with each statement.

The Female Genital Self-Image Scale (FGSIS)

	Strongly Disagree	Disagree	Agree	Strongly Agree
I feel positively about my genitals.	——	——	——	——
I am satisfied with the appearance of my genitals.	——	——	——	——
I would feel comfortable letting a sexual partner look at my genitals.	——	——	——	——
I think my genitals smell fine.	——	——	——	——
I think my genitals work the way they are supposed to work.	——	——	——	——
I feel comfortable letting a healthcare provider examine my genitals.	——	——	——	——
I am not embarrassed about my genitals.	——	——	——	——

Note: Read more about the FGSIS in D. Herbenick, V. Schick, M. Reece, S. Sanders, B. Dodge, and J. D. Fortenberry, "The Female Genital Self-Image Scale (FGSIS): Results from a Nationally Representative Probability Sample of Women in the United States," *Journal of Sexual Medicine* 8, 158–66.

FEMALE GENITAL SELF-IMAGE

In 2010, our research team published two studies in the *Journal of Sexual Medicine* about how women feel about their own genitals, a concept we call "female genital self-image."[30] To measure this

How to score yourself:

1. Give yourself a 1 for each item for which you answered, "Strongly Disagree," a 2 for each item for which you answered "Disagree," a 3 for each "Agree," and a 4 for each "Strongly Agree."
2. Add up your points for a total score (possible points range from 7 to 28).

There is no "right" or "wrong" score on this measure. Women have a wide variety of experiences in their lives that shape how they feel about their genitals. Some women remember being told as little girls not to touch their private parts. They may have been raised to believe that their genitals were dirty or that only "bad girls" touched their privates. As adults, some women are more exposed or susceptible to commercials, such as those for feminine-hygiene products that further suggest that women's genitals are unclean. Other women may have had the very good fortune of having a mother, sister, or good friend teach them about their vulvas and vaginas and let them know that their parts are special, unique, and have the potential for pleasure. Some women first learned to love their bodies, including their genitals, thanks to the appreciative gaze of a loving or lustful partner.

As such, we're not going to take the common approach to self-quizzes that one often finds in women's magazines. As much as we love playing with genital words, we won't tell you, for example, that higher scores make you a "Vulva Vixen" or that certain scores in the lower ranges make you a "Sad Snatch." What we will suggest is that no matter where you fall on the FGSIS, there is always room to rejoice and always room to grow. If you would like to improve how you feel about your genitals, then we hope that this book is a fruitful starting place for you to learn about your body and to embrace it as the wonderful thing that it is.

concept, we created a seven-item scale that women themselves (or doctors, nurses, or researchers) can use—it's called the Female Genital Self-Image Scale, or the FGSIS for short.

In our research, we found that women who engage in health-promoting behaviors, such as having an annual gynecological exam or performing genital self-examination, tend to have a higher female genital self-image.

Curious where you fall? You can take the FGSIS right here in this book (see previous box). And remember: there is no "pass" or "fail" when it comes to FGSIS. Rather, if you find that answering these questions helps you see an area that you'd like to improve on, perhaps you can work on ways to feel better about your genitals.

VULVA AND VAGINA LOVE

All too often we hear negative things about women's genitals: middle-school boys making "vaginas smell like fish" jokes, feminine-hygiene ads that suggest women don't smell "fresh," or advertisements for surgeries that make us question whether we look all right down there. We decided that more women—including us—could benefit from talking about the things they like about their genitals.

In a recent study, we asked women, "What do you like about your genitals?" Hundreds of women responded. Although some women said that they didn't really like their genitals, many were very specific about the things about their lady parts that make them feel happy, aroused, or grateful.

Here is a sampling of what they had to say:

- "They're absolutely beautiful! One labia is slightly longer than the other and folds over the shorter one, and I have slight freckling on my outer labia. They are a wonderful colour, and are very, very responsive."

- "They bring me tremendous pleasure and have participated in giving birth to my two children."
- "That they're my own and unique; that they easily respond to sexual stimulation; that they will one day function in helping to create life; that they look hot; and that they're what make me a woman."
- "I like the look and colour of my labia, the fullness of the outer labia, and the positive way they respond to sexual stimuli."
- "EVERYTHING! The pleasure they bring me, their uniqueness and beauty, their potential for new life (literally and figuratively), their sensual smell, the way they react to stimulation."
- "I like that I am a woman and mine are slightly different from everyone else's. I like that their exact appearance is something I only share with my partner. I think the size/shape/color of every part is just adorable."
- "The uniqueness of the scent. One of my lovers said I smelled earthy and I liked that. I'm also in awe of the way they open up when I'm making love. And I love that my daughter came from them and through them."
- "They bring great sexual pleasure, they feel warm and smooth, they remind me of my womanness, and I really like the smell when I touch myself and bring my finger to my nose."
- "They are strong (I work my Kegel muscles), they are neat and comfortable (I keep the hair trimmed so it doesn't catch on underwear and hurt me), they give me a lot of pleasure with a sexual partner or my vibrators."
- "I have learned to like the appearance of my vulva more so now than when I was younger. I love how I maintain them, Brazilian waxing every six weeks. I actually love that my partner loves my labia."
- "I like the way my genitals look, feel, and smell. I look at my vaginal area often with a mirror, and I do it because I enjoy knowing what it looks like. I also love that it feels so good when touched, and that it helps me have orgasms."

- "I like that they give my husband and me pleasure and that they helped make and deliver my son."
- "Sometimes the smell, I like that guys like them, I like that they give me pleasure, I like that they're mine."
- "I like that they are healthy. I like that they feel good. I like that my inner labia hang down a bit; I think it is mature and sexual. Men like it. I like the colors and textures. I even like the smell."
- "They give me good feelings. They are luscious and voluptuous. They smell and taste good. They birthed a baby."
- "All the different colors (pinks, browns), the shape of the labia, the fluids, the smell, the softness, the pleasure they give me (and sometimes others), one special birthmark."
- "They can be fun to play with."
- "Hmm, haven't really thought about this question before. I guess not much."
- "They're very sensitive! At least the clit is. I like how everything neatly protects itself, like how the labia is all closed up, and then there are flaps over the clit as well. The hair is pretty cool; I've tried different things like shaving and whatnot."
- "Is it bad to say everything about them? I like that I have strawberry blonde pubes—I like the size, length, etc., of my lips, I love my clit and hood (which I want to pierce eventually)."
- "It is very hairy, I like to stroke my genital hair."
- "That they were a part of the creation of my children. That they are unique. That they are powerful."
- "They're very neat 'the perfect pussy' as depicted in porn."
- "They make me feel good they can bring forth life. They are a source of oppression, and while oppression sucks, the fact that so much effort is expended on controlling women's genitals suggests that they're pretty important."
- "I like . . . everything about my genitals? Except maybe that my vagina is quite small so I can't use some of the sex toys I

own—and that's not really something I dislike so much as a vague annoyance. Also, my clitoris is AMAZING. Orgasms—mine being directly related to my genitals—are amazing. I also like how they look, feel, and taste (though I've only been able to taste second-hand), so in short? Everything."

- "Nothing."
- "I like the pleasure they give me. I like the anatomical complexity and the wonder I have from having a clitoris which doesn't seem to have any purpose in the evolutionary sense, but being an organ of pleasure. I like all the orgasms I can have."
- "I like that inside my vulva is red but on the outside it's tones of brown/black. I also like the smell sometimes. I like my genitals a lot when I'm aroused and my pussy lips get all full and plump. I really love how everything down there feels when I'm really wet, like after I've cum. I also like, when my finger is inside myself, to feel myself cum really hard—I really like the feeling of the contractions and the super slick cum."
- "My pubes are awesome and they are very very sensitive, which sometimes I don't like too."
- "I am pretty tight, I like that. I also like that my clit is well hooded and not out in the open. It's wrapped like a present."
- "That they cause such pleasure. I like how it looks. I am very happy with my vagina. Looking forward to pushing a baby out through my vagina someday."

TEST YOUR VQ

1. The inside branches of the clitoris are called
   a. crura
   b. cure-alls
   c. cumulus
   d. coochies

2. The five vaginal shapes are the heart, parallel sides, conical, pumpkin seed, and the
   a. cat
   b. tiger
   c. bee
   d. slug

3. During sexual arousal, a woman's vagina may increase in size due to a process called
   a. vaginal camping
   b. vaginal tenting
   c. vaginal awesomeness
   d. vaginal carousing

Answers

1. a
2. d
3. b

· 2 ·

A Healthy, Happy Vulva

Taking Care Down There

$\mathcal{A}$s children, we learn how to care for our bodies. We learn that exercise is good for our bones, our muscles, and our hearts. Eating fruits and vegetables is good for our bodies as a whole, as they deliver important vitamins and minerals. We also learn about good hygiene: for example, we learn not to pick our nose (at least in public) and that washing hands can prevent colds. And, over time, we learn what's normal about our bodies and what's not. We learn that waking up with sleep in our eyes is a common, healthy occurrence (our eyes need a way to clean themselves out). But we also learn that constant runny noses or coughs are often a sign that we're sick and may need to go to the doctor. We learn these things from our parents and our teachers; perhaps you remember talking about "food groups" in kindergarten or in an elementary school health class. Your physical education teacher may have encouraged you to try running or walking for exercise or to find a sport that you enjoy or are good at. Growing up, we had numerous ways to learn how to care for our bodies and our health.

Curiously, girls and young women learn little about how to care for their genitals beyond the basic potty-training rules of wiping and then washing one's hands. Can you imagine if we women learned information about how to care for our vulvas and vaginas? What if our parents, sisters, or teachers shared information about healthy genital care with girls and young women? What if we could share this information out in the open as if it were just as important as other kinds of health information?

All too often, when girls or women learn how to care for their vulvas and vaginas, it's done with shades of secrecy or taboo. Fifth- and sixth-grade girls are frequently separated from the boys so that they can watch a video about periods and how babies are made (the boys may be outside playing sports or in another room, learning about their own pubertal development). Although there may be some benefits to girls and boys being separated so that they can learn about their sex-specific parts, there may also be some benefit in bringing them together that day, or on another day, to talk and learn about these topics together as a group. After all, boys and girls could benefit from talking with each other about the changes they'll be experiencing over the next few years. Both sexes could learn to talk with respect and compassion about otherwise mysterious topics such as menstruation and erections.

---

9 REASONS TO LOVE YOUR VULVA AND VAGINA

1. It makes it easier to use non-applicator tampons.
2. It makes it easier to use birth-control methods like diaphragms and NuvaRing.
3. It might make you feel more comfortable filming your own birth experience video, should you give birth one day.
4. You may be more comfortable talking with your healthcare provider about your genital health.
5. You may be more open to receiving cunnilingus. Or just plain into it.
6. It could enhance your masturbation to watch yourself in the mirror.
7. Your vagina and vulva will be with you forever, so you may as well make friends.
8. The vagina can be warm and wet to touch, which can feel good.
9. During a self-exam in front of a mirror, it can be fun to make your vulva "talk" by squishing the labia together.

There should be no shame in learning about vulvar and vaginal health. After all, everyone with a vulva and vagina probably wants them to be healthy. Here in this chapter, we'll identify health challenges faced by vulvas and vaginas worldwide and identify key steps that you can take—starting today—toward vulvar and vaginal wellness. That said, we only have room enough to devote one chapter to vulvar and vaginal health issues, so you should consider this a brief overview rather than everything you will ever need to know about genital health. For more extensive information about genital-health issues, we recommend reading *The V Book*[1] (see Resources).

WHAT WE'RE MADE OF

The vulva is a highly sensitive area of women's bodies. Men's genitals are almost completely covered in skin. This skin acts as a protective barrier to the outside world against common irritants and other things that could otherwise harm the genitals. The only opening that men have on their penis is the urethral opening (through which they urinate and ejaculate), and it's a pretty small opening, so not much is going to get through it.

Women, however, have the urethral opening and the vaginal opening, with the latter being significantly larger than the tiny little urethral opening. As such, we're more exposed to the outside world and its many irritants. Also, the vulvar skin is more sensitive and vulnerable to irritation than men's genital skin, so it can be helpful to learn the best way to care for our genital parts. Because genitals and sexual health are such taboo topics in many cultures, many girls and young women don't receive accurate information about how to care for their vulvas and vaginas. It's not necessarily the fault of their mothers, aunts, or grandmothers—after all, many women in older generations never learned much about how to care for their genitals, either. We hope to change that. We hope to give you enough information about how to care for your vulva and vagina so that you feel confident about caring for yourself and sharing this information with your girlfriends as well as with your mom, sister, daughter, niece, grandmother, or neighbor. Even if you don't want to have explicit conversations with friends or family members about v-parts, you can always recommend this or other vulva/vagina-friendly books to them.

VULVA SELF-EXAMINATION: HOW TO CHECK YOURSELF OUT DOWN THERE

One of the simplest and most important ways that you can care for your vulva is to get to know it well. Just as you can care for your skin by checking for suspicious moles or other indications of skin cancer, you can care for your vulva by looking at it about once each month as part of a vulvar self-examination (VSE).

What you will need:

- A well-lit room (if the room's not brightly lit, a flashlight will help)
- A mirror (a self-standing mirror, or one you can lean against the wall, may save you from inverting into some awkward positions)
- Self-love and an open-mind

Here's how:

1. Find at least ten minutes of time when you're unlikely to be interrupted by children, roommates, a partner, the doorbell, or your favorite TV show that's about to come on.
2. In a well-lit room, find a comfortable position in front of your mirror. The angle that you sit at will change the way your vulva appears, so make sure it is a position in which you feel comfortable sitting and exploring. For many women, sitting up

on the bed or against a wall with a pillow behind one's back for comfort or support is a helpful position for VSE.

3. Open your legs enough so that you can clearly see all of your vulva parts.

4. Starting at the top of your genitals (the mons pubis), look at and touch each of your genital parts: the mons, clitoral hood, glans clitoris, labia majora, inner labia, the area around the vaginal entrance, and the perineum. If you are able to view the perianal area (the area around your anus), look at and touch this area as well. Run your fingers through any hair-covered areas so that you can see the skin beneath the hair.

5. Notice what looks and feels normal for you. When you examine your genitals each month, look for any areas that appear to have become darker or lighter, red, itchy, or painful. If you notice any genital changes, discomfort, pain, or new lumps or bumps, ask your healthcare provider about these changes. Chronic itching is also a symptom that should always be brought to the attention of one's healthcare provider.

By performing monthly VSE, you can become familiar with what is normal for your own personal genitals. As every woman is different, this can be an important part of noticing changes that may be related to sexually transmissible infections (such as genital warts), benign skin conditions (such as lichen sclerosus, a skin condition that is often marked by white patches of genital skin), or vulvar cancer that, though rare, has a high survival rate when caught and treated in an early stage. If the size of your genital parts changes, this too is something that you should share with your healthcare provider. Although it's common, for example, for the clitoris to temporarily increase in size when a woman is feeling sexually aroused or after she has just had sex, it is not normal for an adult woman's clitoris to grow substantially bigger (unless she is taking testosterone). In some cases, an enlarged clitoris is a sign of cancer, such as ovarian cancer or adrenal cancer, so it should always be brought to the attention of one's healthcare provider at the earliest opportunity. Or to put it more simply: if your clitoris looks bigger, let your healthcare provider know. Although there are benign reasons for your clitoris to get bigger that have nothing to do with cancer, these are indeed things that should be ruled out. By becoming familiar with your personal "normal" in terms of the shapes, sizes, coloration, and feel of your vulvar parts, you will be better situated to take care of your health and well being.

I really resent that I'm supposed to either fear or love my genitals. They're annoying and frustrating, and I don't feel it's necessary to have strong feelings either way. I am not a bad feminist because I don't love my genitals.

—JAIME, MtF (no surgery), 24, Massachusetts

VULVA AND VAGINA SELF-CARE

Caring for your genital parts involves learning how to tweak some of our most basic daily activities in vulva- and vagina-friendly ways. Here are some tips related to basic hygiene and self-care that can help your lady parts stay happy and healthy.

Wiping

As a child or teenager, you may have been taught to wipe from front to back (the front being toward your clitoris and the back being the anus). Such directions are meant to keep bacteria from the anal opening away from the vagina, as the vagina can be quite sensitive. Generally speaking, it's good advice to wipe from front to back for this reason.

As for what to wipe with, most healthcare providers recommend using regular, unfragranced toilet paper rather than moist wipes (such as those intended for cleaning babies during a diaper change). Moist wipes may have chemicals in them that can irritate the vulvar skin or leave the genitals wet for longer than they need to be. If you prefer to use a moist wipe (some women keep these at home and/or carry these in their purses for wiping when using public bathrooms), ask your healthcare provider to recommend a brand that is unlikely to cause genital irritation when used regularly. Finally, some women use a water bidet to clean after using the bathroom. Patting oneself dry afterward with toilet paper can be helpful, as keeping the genitals wet for too long can cause irritation.

Vaginal Discharge

The uterus, cervix, and vagina produce natural discharge that comes out of the vagina. This is generally called "vaginal discharge" even though the fluids coming out may be coming from the vaginal walls, cervix, or uterus. This is one way in which women's bodies clean themselves. Vaginal discharge is completely natural, and it often changes appearance throughout a woman's menstrual cycle. It may be clear, milky white, or have a slight yellow tinge to it. Sometimes it seems clear and thin. Other times, women notice that their discharge is more clumpy, possibly even leaving little clear or white clumps in their underwear or on the pubic hair closest to their vaginal opening. It's also not uncommon to notice white or light yellow stains on one's underwear. Darker yellow or green discharge or stains may indicate an infection and should be brought to the attention of one's healthcare provider.

If you find that your body produces excessive discharge, we recommend asking your healthcare provider about it. He or she can test you for vaginal infections, including sexually transmissible infections (STIs) that can cause increases in vaginal discharge. After all, some STIs don't have many noticeable symptoms. One woman that Debby knows of noticed that she was experiencing more vaginal wetness than usual, which she attributed to being highly sexually aroused, or horny. When she learned that she had gonorrhea, she was surprised, but it all made sense. This isn't to say that vaginal wetness is always a bad thing (it's not) or that it's never a sign of arousal (often, it is) but if you experience vaginal discharge that is unusual in some way for you, please do bring it to the attention of a healthcare provider. Try to avoid using pantyliners, pads, tampons, or other menstrual products as a way to keep vaginal discharge in check. Menstrual products are only intended for use during a woman's period (i.e., on the days that she is bleeding). Wearing pads or pantyliners too often can irritate the vulva, especially if the pads or pantyliners are fragranced. And wearing tampons on non-period days can make the vagina feel drier and cause irritation as well, so save your period products for your period days! Your body and your wallet will thank you.

Keeping Clean: Easier Than You Think

Because the vagina cleans itself out via vaginal discharge, there's very little to do when it comes to keeping your genital parts clean. However, many women are convinced that they need to clean their lady parts. Here are a few tips to keep in mind:

- **Try to avoid using fragranced and scented bath products.** This includes scented, colored, or antibacterial soaps, as these can irritate the sensitive vulvar skin.
- **Go basic.** Although it surprises some women to hear this, many doctors who specialize in vulvar and vaginal health recommend that women wash their genitals with only water and their hand. That's right: no soaps necessary.
- **Stay soft.** An advantage of using your hand is that it's soft and unlikely to irritate the sensitive genital skin. Loofahs and other cloths meant for scrubbing can irritate the genitals.
- **Avoid soaps.** Harsh soaps and cleansers can cause irritation or itching of the genitals. If you feel you must use some type

of cleanser on your vulva, consider using a gentle cleanser such as Cetaphil (sold over the counter in many drug stores) along with water and your hand.

- **Turn down the heat.** Opt for warm rather than hot showers, as hot water can dry skin all over one's body. Of course, most people opt for warm-to-hot bath water. If you're planning to have sex after a bath, try spending longer than usual in fore-play, as the vagina may be dry (due to the warm water) and may need time to get its lubrication going. You may find it helpful to keep a bottle or packet of personal lubricant nearby in case you need a little assistance with post-bath sex.
- **Don't put any bath products up inside the vagina.** Only the outside parts (the vulva) should be cleaned with water and one's hand. The inside parts (i.e., the vagina) do not require any special cleaning.

Grooming

When grooming your pubic hair, try to choose a kinder, gentler method—something that won't make your genitals run for cover in the other direction. Take care, for example, to groom carefully and not to nick your sensitive, curvy genital parts with razors or scissors. And while we don't think you need pubic hair dye or labia dye, we understand that some women may want to use such products, either to cover gray pubic hairs or to have a little fun with their pubes or labia. We get it. If you go this route, please take care to follow pack-age instructions, to patch test dyes on non-genital parts before using them on genital parts, and to avoid doing anything that doesn't sound right to you. As pubic hair and labia dyes are not approved by any health organization that we know of, the instructions may contain inaccurate information—so please, ask your healthcare provider if you have any questions about whether a product is safe for your cooch or whether you should adjust the instructions in a particular way.

Genital Odor

Most vaginas do not smell like fish—but some do. It is common for women's genitals to have a slight scent to them, sometimes smelling a bit yeasty or like sour milk. This can be normal, healthy, and nothing to worry about. If you have questions about your genital odor, we encourage you to talk with a healthcare provider who can examine you and see if you may have a vaginal infection, such as trichomoniasis, that can result in a strong and often unpleasant odor. In some cases, women may have strong genital odor as a result of overactive sweat glands (this is sometimes treated with Botox). There are tons of sweat glands in the vulva, which is why you may have noticed a damp crotch during exercise. Having sweat glands down there is a good thing. The vulva is full of blood vessels, which means that as blood flow increases to the genital area, it may feel warmer. Sweat allows the warmth to dissipate, which is useful because it will help you feel comfortable as you cool off. In other words, your sweat glands have an important role to play, so try not to be too hard on them.

Douches, Sprays, and Powders

The vagina is a self-cleaning body part. As such, feminine-hygiene products such as douches, deodorant sprays, and powders are not needed to keep the vagina smelling or looking clean (more on this in chapter 5). As this chapter is about health, we'll go a step further and tell you a few additional icky facts about douching: not only can douching not prevent pregnancy or STIs, but douching may make a woman's genital odor and discharge worse instead of better. Why? Because it may promote more bacterial growth. Some research also suggests that women who douche have a greater risk of pelvic inflammatory disease and of ectopic pregnancy, which is when a pregnancy begins to develop outside of the uterus (such as in the fallopian tube). Bottom line: avoid these kinds of feminine hygiene products unless specifically recommended by a healthcare provider.

What to Wear Down There

As the vulva can be quite sensitive, healthcare providers sometimes suggest that the most vagina/vulva-friendly underwear is cotton underwear, as it allows the genitals to "breathe." It also helps to keep the genital area dry rather than trapping moisture.

Some women also find it helpful or comfortable to sleep or go through their day without wearing underwear. This may be particularly helpful if they are prone to genital discomfort or pain. In addition, thong underwear has been identified as a common irritant of the vulva, so you may find it more comfortable to choose other styles of underwear.

Laundry

Although most women find that they can use any laundry detergent they want and not experience genital irritation, not all women are so lucky. If you're prone to vaginal or vulvar irritation, itching, or pain, you may want to use a detergent that is free of fragrances and dyes. Some women even run their laundry—or at least their underwear—through an additional rinse cycle to further dilute any detergent that may be lingering in their undies.

EXERCISE

Exercise and Clothing

Not only is regular physical exercise good for the heart, lungs, weight management, and overall wellness, it can also feel invigorating for many women. Plus, exercise helps many women to manage menstrual or premenstrual symptoms such as cramps and irritability.

If you exercise (and we hope you do, whether it's walking, running, swimming, dancing, or taking your dog out for long walks), try to change out of your exercise clothes or underwear soon after you're done exercising. This can help to keep your genitals dry rather than having them trapped with all that moisture from sweating, which can irritate the genitals. Putting on clean, dry clothes is a welcome relief for vulvas and vaginas worldwide.

Heave, Ho

When you lift objects, try to adopt a healthy lifting posture (you know, the whole "bend at the knees" thing). It's not just good for your back, but it might be vagina-friendly, too. Why? Because the pelvic-floor muscles support the bottoms of our bodies including our vaginas, rectums, and reproductive organs. Lifting heavy things, especially improperly, can put strain on the pelvic-floor muscles and weaken them over time. Body weight, including weight gained during pregnancy or even when one is not pregnant, can also put strain on the pelvic-floor muscles. Of course, it's important to be open to gaining a healthy amount of weight during pregnancy but that amount varies from woman to woman. If you are pregnant or thinking about becoming pregnant, ask your OB/GYN for advice about attaining a healthy pregnancy, including a healthy pregnancy weight. And if you are not pregnant but have questions about your health, weight, or body composition, your healthcare provider can be a good source of information as can a registered dietician. (Note: an RD is different from a "nutritionist," which anyone can call himself or herself, even with no advanced training.)

Kegels

Kegel (say "kay-gull") exercises are named for the gynecologist Dr. Arnold Kegel who first described these exercises as a way to help women maintain bladder control. Just as certain exercises can help to strengthen leg muscles or arm muscles, Kegel exercises can help to improve the tone of the pelvic-floor muscles. This can be important in terms of helping to reduce the risk of incontinence that otherwise increases with age and childbearing. Some women feel that pelvic-floor exercises also help them to experience more intense orgasms, though this is not well understood in research.

To identify your pelvic-floor muscles, try stopping the flow of urine as you pee. Those are the muscles that—when you're not peeing—you will want to squeeze as part of your Kegel exercises. Another way to identify these muscles is by inserting a finger into the vagina and squeezing the muscles, which will likely result in a sense of pressure around the finger. Sex educators and healthcare providers often recommend different variations on Kegel exercises. For example, they may recommend that women:

- Squeeze the pelvic-floor muscles and hold to the count of five, then release for another five counts. Repeat the squeeze-and-release pattern for five minutes. Eventually work up to ten minutes.
- Squeeze and release the pelvic-floor muscles in a quick pulsing pattern, squeezing for only one or two seconds and then releasing for the same. Try to do this for up to five minutes.
- Use a Kegel exerciser as part of the exercises. A Kegel exerciser often looks like a small, thin, weighted bar (about the length of a typical dildo, or smaller). Some women insert the weighted bar an inch or two into their vagina as they practice their preferred squeeze/release pattern. Over time, some women begin inserting more of the weighted bar into their vagina so that it holds more weight. Using water-based lubricant can help to make it easier to insert the weighted bar into the vagina. Also make sure to clean the bar before and after use.
- Use balls meant for Kegel exercises, such as Ben Wa balls or Smart Balls, as part of one's Kegel exercises. Some women opt to place one ball inside their vagina and use it to squeeze and then relax their muscles. Others opt to place two balls inside

the vagina as part of their Kegel exercises. Another variation is to place one or both balls inside the vagina, squeeze one's pelvic-floor muscles, and then walk several feet or the full length of one's room using only the strength of one's pelvic-floor muscles to keep the ball(s) inside the vagina. Again, water-based lubricant can help to make insertion more comfortable, and cleaning the balls before and after use is recommended. These balls can be found in many of the sex shops listed in the Resources section.

While practicing Kegel exercises, try to focus only on the pelvic-floor muscles by lifting up rather than bearing down or using other nearby muscles, such as the abdominal muscles. Try to find a time when you are relaxed, comfortable, and have sufficient time to complete your exercises without interruption. Some women do their Kegel exercises daily, and others aim for a few times per week. If you have any questions or concerns about how to perform Kegel exercises or if they are right for you, please check in with your healthcare provider, as everyone's body and personal-health needs are a little different. Women who experience genital pain, including pain during sex, are particularly encouraged to seek advice from their healthcare provider, such as a physical therapist who has experience treating women for genital-pain issues, prior to starting a program of pelvic-floor exercises like Kegels. This is because some women with a genital-pain disorder may have pelvic-floor muscles that are too tight, and they may benefit from different kinds of exercises.

DITCH THE ITCH

One of the most common complaints that women have about their genitals has to do with itching. On the plus side, this means that you can pretty much always find a shoulder to lean on when it comes to genital itching. If you mention it to a friend or to your mom, chances are she's been there, too. On the down side, this also means that itching is a non-specific symptom. If your vulva itches, it doesn't exactly narrow down the list of many things that could be causing the itching. That said, there are a few common causes of genital itching among women. The next time you feel all "ugh!" down there, consider whether any of these may be at the root of your problem:

- **Clothing.** We've said it before, and we'll say it again. Women's genitals do not like to be bound up and restricted. Multiple layers (think pantyliner, tights, and a skirt) or too-tight clothes, such as spandex pants or tight jeans, can trap moisture. These kinds of clothes can be fine on occasion, but if you opt to spend the day in leggings, try to air out your bits by sleeping in the nude, or at least going without panties, at night. Let your vulva and vagina breathe! Truly, you may be surprised by how many cases of genital itching could be prevented by wearing fewer layers, loose cotton underwear, or more natural, breathable fabrics. Try not to wear constrictive pantyhose or "shape" products (e.g., Spanx) too often.
- **Chemical irritants.** You may not think twice about pouring bleach in the laundry, but that bleach may be irritating your lady bits. And if your male partner is using performance-enhancing condoms that help him to last longer, then your itching may be linked to the benzocaine or lidocaine that's in some of those products. Or if you have ever thought it would be a good idea to sanitize your menstrual cup or sponge with tea tree oil, think again—that, too, can irritate women's sensitive genitals. There have even been case reports of women experiencing genital irritation from newspaper ink.[2] That's right—newspaper ink. It turns out that their partners were reading the newspaper in bed before sex. The ink got on their hands, and their hands got on their partner's genitals, and next thing you know, there's a case of mysteriously irritated genitals. If your bed partner reads the newspaper before bed,

ask him or her to wash up before going any further. (Perhaps this is yet another reason why digital newspapers are a good option!)

- **Bath products.** Although these probably belong in the "chemical irritant" section, bath products are so commonly linked to genital itching and irritation that they deserve their own mention. Women's vaginal itching and irritation are commonly linked to fragranced products, and bath products are among the worst culprits.[2] Although these products may help create a relaxing, fragrant retreat out of your shower or bath, women find themselves less relaxed later when their bits begin to itch. If you choose to use fancy schmancy bath products anyway, try to use only a small amount and dilute them greatly with bath water.

- **Your lubricant.** Although lubricant formulations are getting better every day, many lubricants that you'll find on store shelves contain propylene glycol or chlorhexidine, which have also been linked to genital itching or irritation among women.[1] If you notice ongoing itching, check the labels of your lubricants and consider switching products.

- **Feminine hygiene products.** Please forgive us for saying this over and over again, but feminine hygiene products such as douches, sprays, and deodorants can cause more harm than good. And they can definitely contribute to vulvar itching for some women.

- **Yogurt.** Although Debby's refrigerator is constantly stocked with dozens of cups of yogurt, her vagina is not. You won't find any yogurt near our lady parts. Why? Because it doesn't belong there. Forget what you may have read on the Internet about using yogurt down there to fight yeast infections. The next time you have an urge to put food of any kind on or in your genitals, check with your healthcare provider first, as even food—particularly when misplaced—can cause vulvar itching or irritation.

- **Yeast infections.** Many women feel itchy down there and race to the drug store to get over-the-counter yeast medications. This can be a huge mistake. Why? Well, if you don't have a yeast infection, then not only will yeast creams not work, but they may also make your itching and other genital symptoms worse. Or, equally bad is that the cream and any side effects you have from the cream may make it more difficult for your healthcare provider to properly diagnose the cause of your genital symptoms. As such, we recommend always checking in with your healthcare provider before seeking help from over-the-counter yeast infection medications. One of the few exceptions to this is that women who are super prone to yeast infections (meaning, they get four or more per year) are probably pretty good at telling what is and what is not a yeast infection due to experience. Some healthcare providers tell these women that they can probably make the yeast-cream decision on their own without much risk. But if you're not sure, or if you have questions about your personal health, definitely check in with your healthcare provider. If you do have a yeast infection, your healthcare provider can walk you through your treatment options, which may include over-the-counter yeast cream, a prescription pill, or other treatments if the yeast is an uncommon type that doesn't respond to typical treatments.

- **Medications.** Sometimes women's healthcare providers advise them to use over-the-counter or prescription creams on their genitals, for example, to treat skin disorders (such as lichen sclerosus) or STIs (such as genital warts). Yeast creams, estrogen or testosterone creams, and even numbing agents may be used on the genital skin, or internally, for different reasons, per the advice of one's healthcare provider. Occasionally, women experience itching, irritation, or feelings of burning, stinging, or pain when they use such creams. If your healthcare provider prescribes a cream or ointment for you to use on your vulva or inside your vagina, ask him or her what kinds of symptoms you can expect and what to do if you experience them (e.g., Stop the medication? Press an ice pack against your vulva to stop the pain?).

SEXY TIMES

It's common for women and men to incorporate sexual-enhancement products into their sex lives. Using sex toys, creams, or lubricants can add novelty to a relationship, be a fun part of sex play, or help to make sex feel more comfortable, romantic, sexy, or more easily orgasmic. However, many sex toys don't come with instructions for safe or plea-surable use—let alone vagina-friendly instructions. To make the most of your sexual experiences, consider the following:

I wish girls were taught from younger ages the correct names for all body parts, and empowered to love their genitals. I wish there was continued movement away from vaginal orgasms being the "preferred" kind.

—ELIZABETH, 41, Michigan

- **Clean any sex toys before and after you use them.** After cleaning them, air dry your sex toys before putting them away so that they're not kept in a warm, moist environ-ment, which can encourage bacterial growth.
- **Take care with a condom.** If you're prone to vulvar or vaginal irritation, or if your vibrator or dildo is made of a soft, porous material (such as Jelly), consider slipping a new condom over the vibrator or dildo before inserting it into your vagina. This is a definite must if you are sharing a vi-brator or dildo with one or more partners or friends (not recommended, though we realize people do it anyway).

- **Avoid douching, unless recommended by a healthcare provider.** Douching after sex does not prevent pregnancy, and it can disrupt the otherwise friendly vaginal environment.
- **If you enjoy bathing alone or with a partner before sex, consider steering clear of bubble baths, as they may irritate the vulva or vagina.** Instead, add a few drops of an essential oil to the bath. Alternatively, you might find that lighting scented candles in the bathroom adds to the sensuality of the bath experience without increasing your risk of genital irritation.
- **Choose a vagina-friendly lubricant.** In other words, one without propylene glycol, chlorhexidine, or other chemicals that you may be sensitive or allergic to (you may not be sensitive to the two we listed, but some women find that they contribute to genital irritation). If you're trying to conceive, consider a lubricant such as Pre-Seed that is unlikely to interfere with sperm movement.
- **Examine your birth control.** Spermicidal products, such as spermicidal foams and jellies, irritate some women's vaginas. Some women who experience chronic vulvar or vaginal pain have been advised by their healthcare providers to switch methods of birth control. If you have ongoing issues of vulvar or vaginal discomfort or pain, talk with your healthcare provider about the current method of contraception you are using and whether another method may be a better choice for you.
- **Go plain.** Although flavored lubricants can seem fun, they're not for everyone. Keep in mind that men's and women's genitals are quite different from each other. Because men's genitals are mostly covered with skin, men can often more easily tolerate flavored and sugary products on their genitals. Similar products can cause irritation on lady parts. As such, opt for plain lubricants over flavored lubricants, sprinkle body sugar or spread body frosting on your breasts or stomach (rather than

your vulva), and use flavored condoms for oral sex only. Flavored condoms can cause irritation if used vaginally.

- **Wash him off.** Be sure to wash any sugars, body frosting, or flavored lubricant off of your partner's penis (if male) or your sex toy before you allow it to enter into your vagina. Flavored, sugary sex-play products can be fun and tasty, but they don't belong in your vagina and may cause vaginal itching or irritation. Run a small washcloth under warm water and then use it to clean his penis before you go further into the Land of Penetrative Sex. The same is true if you have a female or male partner wearing or using a strap-on/dildo: if you've made it tasty for oral-sex play, clean it before it goes back inside your body.

- **Lower your yeast risk.** Although it can feel pleasurable to receive oral sex, it's not for everyone—and not just because of personal preference. Some women are particularly prone to recurrent yeast infections. Research suggests that these women may face an increased risk of yeast infections if they have intercourse with a male partner who has saliva on his penis (for example, if she or he put saliva on his penis as a lubricant, or if she recently performed oral sex on him).[3] Women are also more prone to repeat yeast infections if they frequently received oral sex from a partner. If you're prone to repeat yeast infections, you might find it helpful to meet with a vulvovaginal specialist (find one through issvd.org or nva.org). You might also find it helpful to use a dental dam or condom cut in half during cunnilingus or to wash his penis or your toy off before intercourse.

PERIOD DOS AND DON'TS

Most women experience menarche between the ages of ten and fourteen and reach menopause by their early fifties. Women in the United

States and many Western countries don't tend to have large numbers of children. This means that women will commonly spend three to four decades of their lives having monthly (or thereabouts) periods. Whether you started menstruating last month or twenty years ago, you can benefit from the health-related period tips in this section.

Women have a wide variety of period products to choose from including tampons, pads, pantyliners, menstrual cups, and menstrual sponges. Most women can use any of these without upsetting the vulva or vagina goddesses. Others have to choose more carefully based on their own health needs. We describe all of the products in detail in chapter 5, but here are a few things to consider when pondering the impact of period products on your health:

Tampons

Tampons are one of the most popular methods of period management among women in the United States. But that doesn't mean that women can't benefit from being reminded about how to use them for the safest possible experience. First and foremost, let's start with a few tips on the greatest danger associated with tampons: TSS.

What's TSS? It stands for toxic shock syndrome. If you have never known anyone who has ever had it, you are in good company. At the height of the TSS scare, only thirty-five people were diagnosed with it (and ten of those people were men). Of the women, the majority had vaginal symptoms, which suggested it was related to menstruation.[4] Then, in 1980, use of a certain super-absorbency tampon was found to be linked to TSS. Hence, the association with tampons. The tampons that were linked with TSS risk were quickly taken off the market, and the FDA has done a fine job of monitoring the market since then. TSS in connection with period products still occurs, but it is extremely rare. There is approximately one case of TSS out of every one hundred thousand menstruating women per year.[4] That isn't 1 percent—not even .1 percent or .01 percent. Only .001 percent of women have been diagnosed with TSS.

So, what's with the scary warning on your tampon packages/instructions? Although it is unlikely that you will get TSS, if you do, it can have some very serious health consequences including shock, liver and kidney failure, and possibly even death if left untreated. If you think you have it, don't panic! Over 95 percent of women will recover from it, which are some pretty good odds.[4] Still, as with most things, TSS gets worse the longer it goes untreated. So, to be on the safe side, take out your tampon and consult a doctor if you have the following symptoms:[4]

- a fever over 102 degrees
- a rash (it may appear to look like sunburn)
- vomiting or diarrhea
- disorientation
- muscle aches
- red eyes
- fainting from a sudden drop in blood pressure

In addition to being aware of the symptoms, you can reduce your risk by taking a few extra precautions. First, always try to choose the tampon with the lowest absorbency necessary to get the job done. Researchers are mixed on how much this actually matters, with one study finding that there really are no notable safety differences between ultra- and super-plus-absorbency tampons.[5] Although these absorbencies don't even sound that different, we still recommend this because it is better to be safe than sorry, and it just seems like a good general rule to use as little absorbency as needed. Besides, it can be uncomfortable to insert a large tampon without the proper lubrication!

That brings us to rule number 2: Change your tampon often in accordance with the recommendations listed on the tampon package insert or from your healthcare provider. Tampons that are left too long inside the vagina can cause bacterial infections or, although rare, can increase the risk of TSS. We know it's easier on you and the bank account to leave the tampon in until it feels ready to pop, but it is better to follow the guidelines and change them every few hours. Following these steps can help to reduce the risk of TSS, which, although rare, can be deadly.

In addition to TSS, we've seen some scary emails floating around the cyber universe that make it seem as though regular tampons will cause all sorts of health problems (for example, that they contain asbestos). We know of no evidence that supports these claims. In fact, the US Food and Drug Administration (FDA) issued a statement in 1999 indicating that it had "no evidence of asbestos in tampons."[6] And given the choice between believing the FDA or emails that also claim to come from foreigners who want to transfer millions of US dollars into your bank account, we'll believe the FDA.

Menstrual Pads and Pantyliners

It is recommended that women only use menstrual pads or pantyliners on days that they are menstruating. If you find that you experience excessive vaginal discharge and want to use pads or liners for this reason, consider checking in with a healthcare provider before doing so. As we've mentioned, using pads or liners too often can cause or contribute to genital itching, redness, and/or irritation.

Sex and Your Period

Although some women avoid having sex while on their period, others are quite happy to have sex with a partner while menstruating. For some women, sexual pleasure and orgasm seem to help with any period-related discomfort, such as cramps. Also, some women find that they're highly aroused while menstruating. If you want to have sex while menstruating, it is a perfectly common thing to do—and it is not "unhealthy." Of course, any time there is exposure to blood there may be a greater risk of infection, so you'll want to make sure to use a condom and/or talk with your partner about each of your STI histories. A tip: some people find it helpful to lay a towel down

on the bed or other area (floor?) where they plan to have sex to reduce the likelihood of staining one's sheets.

BIRTH CONTROL

Women and men commonly have questions about birth control.
They want to know how effective different types of birth control
are, how much they cost, and how easy they are to use. Perhaps
you've also wondered how certain birth-control methods interact
with your precious v-parts, the vulva and vagina. Given the dozens
of different types of birth control available, we don't have room to
go over every single one here. However, this brief overview of common birth-control methods and how they relate to your vulva and
vagina, or your sex life, should be a good start:

Male Condoms

Most women who have male sexual partners find that male condoms
are incredibly vagina-friendly. After all, male condoms—when used
correctly and consistently, and when they stay intact (which they
nearly always do)—keep semen away from the vagina, thus reducing
the risk of infection and unintended pregnancy. That's pretty vagina-
friendly, if you ask us! Every now and then, though, women will say
that they feel irritated after having sex with a condom-clad partner.
If you are sensitive or allergic to latex condoms, choose condoms
made of something other than latex, such as polyurethane. Even if
you're not sensitive or allergic to condoms, you may find that your
vagina and vulva are more comfortable when you use a certain brand
of condom. It's possible that you may be reacting to the lubricant on
the condom, if it's pre-lubricated. Make note of condoms that work
particularly well with your body and keep some on hand so that
you'll be ready to have safer sex.

Female Condoms

American women rarely use female condoms; they are more commonly used by women and promoted by health groups in other countries. Female condoms look like pouches. The closed end is inserted head first into the vagina with the outer edges folding over the vulva. Some women find that using a female condom gives them more control over having safer sex. Condom-using couples may find this a fun, pleasurable, and safe (albeit sometimes expensive) way to diversify their sex lives.

NuvaRing

The NuvaRing is a vaginal-ring contraceptive. Women only need to insert one ring into the vagina and then leave it there for three weeks. Some women worry that leaving the NuvaRing in the vagina for three weeks is unhealthy for the vagina. It's not (that is, assuming the ring stayed in its original packaging and then a woman washed her hands before opening the package, removing the ring, and inserting it into her vagina). Women also sometimes wonder if male partners will feel the NuvaRing during sex. In one study of women using NuvaRing and their partners, nearly 70 percent of men said that they never felt the ring during sex (it's inserted pretty far up the vagina).[7] Those who do feel the NuvaRing don't, for the most part, appear to be bothered by it. However, every woman is built differently, and every couple has bodies that fit together differently and different ways of having sex, including favorite or go-to sex positions. If you try the NuvaRing and find it's uncomfortable for either one of you during sex, you may be able to remove it during sex (but not for long—ask your healthcare provider for details), as long as you remember to reinsert it soon afterward. Otherwise, consider other birth-control options that may be a better fit for you.

Birth-Control Pills

Birth-control pills are widely used by women around the world. Some women who take low-dose estrogen pills notice that they lubricate less than they used to (estrogen plays a role in vaginal lubrication). Also, keep in mind that birth-control pills are to be taken orally, meaning swallowed by mouth. We mention this only because every now and then, we hear about women who mistakenly believe that birth-control pills work by inserting them into the vagina. This is not the case! Please do NOT insert your birth-control pills into your (or anyone else's) vagina. If you have questions about how to take birth-control pills or any other medication, please check in with your healthcare provider.

Diaphragms

Diaphragms are less commonly used in the United States, but they are still an important barrier method of birth control, meaning they help keep semen from reaching the cervix, uterus, and fallopian tubes. Women who use diaphragms appear to be at increased risk of urinary tract infections (UTI), which are infections of the urethra, bladder, the tubes that connect the bladder to the kidneys, or the kidneys themselves.[8] Any time you suspect that you may have a UTI, it's worth checking in with a healthcare provider who can advise you on possible home treatment and/or prescription treatment.

Cervical Caps

Cervical caps fit over the cervix, thus serving as a barrier to keep sperm away from the cervix, uterus, and fallopian tubes (just like diaphragms and condoms, in this regard). If you've had a baby since you last used a cervical cap, check in with your healthcare provider, as you may need to be re-fitted for one.

Spermicides

Spermicides may come in foams, jellies, or films. Spermicidal lubricant may also be used on male condoms. Although many women tolerate spermicide just fine, some women experience vulvovaginal irritation, such as vaginal burning, itching, or pain, when they use spermicidal products. If you experience genital irritation, we recommend asking your healthcare provider for recommendations about birth-control methods that may be a better fit for your vaginal and vulvar health.

WHAT TO EXPECT WHEN YOU'RE EXPECTING (TO GO TO THE GYNECOLOGIST)

Going to the gynecologist. Whether you love or hate it, the American College of Obstetricians and Gynecologists (ACOG) recommends that all women—even women who are not sexually active or who are past their childbearing years—go to the gynecologist. Nervous? Try not to be. We'll give you all the information you need to prepare yourself or someone else for a visit to the gynecologist, whether it's your first time ever or your first time in a long time.

When Should I Go?

As we said previously, the most recent guidelines recommend that young women have their first appointment with a gynecologist between the ages of thirteen and fifteen, though not necessarily for a pelvic exam or Pap test (those often come later; in fact, at this writing, Pap tests are recommended for most women beginning at the age of twenty-one).

Where Should I Go?

If you feel comfortable discussing it with your mother/female care-giver/relative/teacher, they will likely be able to provide you with a good local recommendation. With over eight hundred health centers across the United States, you are also bound to find a Planned Parenthood near you (see Resources). The nice thing about Planned Parenthood is that they do their best to provide affordable care for everyone. This means that you do not need health insurance or permission from a parent, in most cases, in order to schedule a visit.

I once had an amazingly considerate female gynaecologist who asked about my sexual experiences before examining me, took them into consideration with the diagnosis and was so careful when examining me that although my health issues have not [ever] been resolved and probably never will be, that consultation stands out as the most positive doctor's experience I have ever had. I think all gynae-cologists should be trained like she was. I can't stress enough how much better I felt about my body and my health after seeing her.

—Josie, 26, United Kingdom

How Do I Prepare for My Visit?

There is not much that you need to do before you visit the gyne-cologist other than trying to schedule an appointment during a time when you are not menstruating. Other than that, there are a few things that you should try *not* to do. You should try to refrain from having unprotected vaginal intercourse for a day or two before your exam. If you douche, it is best not to douche within the week before your appointment. Also, try to stay away from using vaginal wipes, foams, and sprays during the week before your visit. All of these things may make it more difficult to interpret your Pap test results.

What Happens during the Exam?

- Prior to meeting with your healthcare provider, you will be asked to fill out a comprehensive medical history. Try not to let shyness or embarrassment get in the way of reporting your sexual or health history. Also, be sure to list all of your genital symptoms (e.g., itching, burning, pain). Providers need accurate information in order to make informed decisions about your health. If this is your first visit, or if you're nervous or scared, you may want to indicate that on the paperwork or tell the nurse during the initial intake.

- Prior to beginning the exam, your healthcare provider will hopefully take some time to talk with you about your history and what you should expect from your visit. This is a great time to ask lots of questions. Some clinics will automatically test you for STIs, while others will not, so be sure to ask. By asking questions, you will be informed about what is going to happen, and your healthcare provider will have the information necessary to tailor the exam in ways that will maximize your comfort and health. If you feel more comfortable, you can have a family member, friend, or partner stay in the exam room with you.

- After answering your questions, your healthcare provider will likely bring you to a private space where you will be provided with a paper or cloth gown to change into. Some gowns are made differently than others, so don't be afraid to ask how to put it on.

- If these have not already been done during the intake, the exam will begin as most doctors' visits do: measuring your height, weight, blood pressure, etc. Next, the provider will likely begin with a breast exam to look for any tumors. You will probably be asked to lift one hand up as the provider feels for tumors in your breasts. After your breast exam, the provider will likely feel your abdomen for pain or other indications of abnormalities.

- Finally, you will be asked to move toward the edge of the exam table and place your feet in stirrups in order to provide an ample view of your vulva and vagina. Your provider will begin by doing an external exam of your genitals in order to check your vulvar skin, examine any discharge, or look for potential abnormalities. Next, your provider will insert a lubricated speculum (it looks a little like a duck's bill) into your vagina in order to separate the walls of the vagina so that he/she can view your cervix and swab it quickly with a long cotton swab (similar to a Q-tip). This is done to test for cervical changes and may also be used to test for some infections. This is not painful for most women. If it is for you, make sure to tell your healthcare provider because the solution may be as simple as using a speculum of another size. After your speculum exam, your provider may insert one or two lubricated fingers into your vagina while pressing down on your abdomen. This is done to check for potential issues with your uterus or fallopian tubes. Then, your provider may conduct a rectovaginal exam by inserting a single lubricated finger into your anus and one into your vagina in order to check for tumors behind the rectum or the lower wall of the vagina. After the exam is done, your healthcare provider may ask you to change back into your clothes while he or she leaves the room. When he or she returns, you may have the chance to talk more about the exam, to ask additional questions, and to further talk about your personal health.

A few tips:

1. If you want to see your vulva and cervix, ask your practitioner to hand you a mirror. It can be fun and informative!

2. If you are nervous during the exam, give your provider a few
   tips about the best ways to help you relax. Do you want up-
   to-the-minute details on what he/she is doing? Perhaps you
   would prefer to be distracted by some small talk? It is best for
   you, your provider, and your health if you are relaxed, so
   speak up!

That's it; all done! Now that wasn't so bad—was it?

RAISING A DAUGHTER

When women finally learn about their vulvas and vaginas, they are
often well into adulthood. We envision a future in which more parents feel comfortable and confident taking care of their young
daughter's genital health and raise them with correct information as
soon as they begin teaching them to speak. If you are raising a
daughter or are otherwise caring for a young girl, we hope that this
information will be helpful to you:

**Although very rare, it is possible for a girl to be born
without a vagina or with a very small vagina.** In many
cases, a vagina can be surgically created when she is older
(genital surgeries are only very rarely recommended for babies
or young children, such as in cases where they are medically
necessary).

Her clitoris may appear unusually large. When a baby is first
born, she has estrogen from her mother's blood supply. As estrogen is linked to a range of vaginal and vulvar features, this
means that she will likely experience vaginal lubrication and
discharge during the first few weeks of life. Her labia majora
and minora may also be noticeably plump. After several weeks,
when she no longer is impacted by her mother's estrogen, her
mons and outer labia will likely shrink in size. This may make

her clitoris and inner labia look larger than before, but that is a normal occurrence. Girls often "grow into" their genitals around the time of puberty. However, if you have any questions about your daughter's genital size, ask her pediatrician.

Even a baby may experience vaginal bleeding. When a baby no longer has her mother's estrogen supply, her uterus may shed some of its lining due to the drop in estrogen levels. As such, some female babies experience small amounts of vaginal bleeding during their first few weeks of life outside the womb.

Her labia may stick together. Without her mother's estrogen supply, a baby or toddler's inner labia may stick together, a condition called "labial adhesion." In the United States, it happens to about 2 percent of female babies and children up to the age of six.[9] The inner labia may stick together just a little or a lot, covering some or much of the vaginal opening or urethra (which can be problematic in terms of having urine pool there). If you have a daughter and notice this when changing her diaper or helping her go to the bathroom, you should mention it to her pediatrician. Sometimes no treatment is needed and the inner labia separate on their own. Other times, an estrogen cream is prescribed, and a girl's parents or caretakers are asked to apply it to her labia, often for a matter of weeks. The cream often helps the labia to separate. In rare cases, if the cream is ineffective (as it is for approximately 20 to 50 percent of girls), a quick surgical procedure should permanently resolve the problem.[10–12] It is not usually an ongoing medical problem, but it is something to speak with one's pediatrician about.

She may touch herself. Young babies, both male and female, often touch their genitals. Then again, they touch many of their body parts. This is not unusual. Studies of parents and caregivers indicate that the vast majority of young children touch their own genitals. Many children, as we'll discuss later, also play games that involve comparing their private parts.

This is also common and a normal part of exploration. Some children touch their genitals with their fingers. Others stimulate their genitals by rubbing their bodies against toys, bedding, pillows, stuffed animals, or the floor. Many pediatricians and child psychologists recommend that parents respond in a way that assures their child that touching one's genitals is okay and that their genitals are not dirty. For example, a parent might say something like, "That's okay to do, but please do it somewhere private, such as in your bedroom or in the bathroom." Of course, this may be more appropriate for older children (often aged four and up) who can understand the message.

Vaginal insertion. Some young girls insert objects into their vaginas for reasons that are unclear. One mother, whose daughter was found to have inserted part of a Bratz doll into her vagina, wondered if perhaps her daughter had seen her insert a tampon and tried to imitate this action with her toy.[13] For other young girls, the vaginal insertion of objects may be linked to sexual abuse. Other times, girls may have just found their vagina one day, inserted a finger, and then wondered what else could be placed in their "special hiding place." For some, inserting toys or objects into the vagina may be a form of self-stimulation. Mostly, though, we just don't know why some young girls do this, as research has largely been focused on taking care of these girls' health needs. When you teach your daughter about her genitals, it is worth teaching her how to care for them, including that her vagina is not a place to keep things. We say this only half-jokingly, as it cannot be emphasized enough that there are dangers associated with girls putting objects into the vagina and leaving them there. Some girls who have had ongoing fevers and/or abdominal pain were eventually brought to the emergency room, only to find that they had inserted batteries into the vagina.[14, 15] These have resulted in serious health emergencies, very careful removal by skilled physicians, and (in some cases) hospitalization.

V-CRAFT: HOST YOUR OWN "DINNER PARTY"!

A vulva-themed party can be fun to host for no other reason than to celebrate our down theres—and what better way to name it than your own "Dinner Party" in honor of Judy Chicago's famous vulva-themed art installation (more on this later)? If you're the kind of person who likes to party with purpose, why not host a vulva-themed party as a fundraiser for your local V-Day cast and crew's production of *The Vagina Monologues*? Or donate the proceeds to the National Vulvodynia Association? Or host in recognition of International GYN Awareness Day (IGAD), celebrated on September 10 or in recognition of Vulvar Health Awareness Month, celebrated each March? Here are some ideas:

1. Make vulva-themed cupcakes by using frosting to draw vulvas or the letter "V" on each cupcake (we recommend frosting some in pink, others in beige or brown or black, and others in red or purple, etc).
2. Entertain yourselves by playing pin the clitoris on the vulva! Draw your own poster-sized vulva, equipped with all its parts, and cheer each other on as partygoers put the clitoris in its rightful place.
3. Make vulva-themed plates in advance, perhaps at your local paint-your-own-pottery place. In our experience, we were not censored—then again, the vulvas we've made on plates have been a bit Georgia O'Keeffe-ish, in that they looked as much like flowers as they did vulvas.
4. Give out hand mirrors as party favors along with information about vulvar self-examination.
5. Color your vulvas! Set out crayons and pages from the *Cunt Coloring Book* and get together and draw your own or your imaginary vulvas.

Use your imagination to make this a vulva-positive evening full of good friends, food, and energy.

Give her the words. When you teach your daughter the names for her body parts, try to teach her the words she will need to talk about and think about her genital body parts. Just as she should know words for her elbows, cheeks, chest, and legs, we feel that young girls should also know the words vulva, vagina, and labia, among others. In her sex-education work, Debby has given puberty talks to a number of girls and their moms (as well as boys and their dads). In these conversations, she has been able to teach girls the names of all their vulva parts, including the clitoris, urethral opening, outer labia, and inner labia. The girls have often been happy to learn that they have a body part that is just about sensation and feeling good (that's right: without giving them more detail than they may be ready for, it is possible to teach even young girls about the clitoris and its purpose related to pleasure). They're also often very curious to learn about periods in the years approaching puberty, and having a good sense of the uterus, cervix, and vagina can help them to have more clear conversations with their moms, aunts, sisters, girlfriends, teachers, healthcare providers, or other adult caregivers.

If she itches, get her help. Because young girls lack estrogen before puberty, they rarely have many vaginal problems, such as yeast infections. However, that doesn't mean that nothing will ever bother her vagina. If a girl experiences ongoing vaginal itching, she may have a skin disorder affecting her genitals called lichen sclerosus. It can affect babies, children, or adults. Treatment (usually by a topical steroid cream) can often relieve symptoms, such as itching. Unfortunately, some healthcare providers are not familiar with this health condition and may mistakenly wonder if the girl has been sexually abused (sometimes genital symptoms are indeed a sign of sexual abuse). Itching can also be caused by bath products, such as bubble baths, which should be limited during childhood along with staying in a wet bathing suit or exercise clothes too long or not wiping after urinating.

Raising children or otherwise caring for them—whether as a parent, aunt, uncle, babysitter, or teacher—is important work. For more information about books on how to talk to children and teenagers about sexuality and genital-health issues, see the Resources section where we also list books for children to read by themselves or together with a parent or caregiver.

Get her GYN care. As girls become teenagers, it can be helpful to get them started with gynecological care. The ACOG recommends that sometime between the ages of thirteen and fifteen, young women can benefit from having their first gynecological exam if they haven't yet had one. Depending on a young woman's personal health needs, this first visit may only include conversation about menstruation and pubertal changes. The visit may simply help to get her comfortable with her gynecologist and the idea of a future gynecological exam. Then again, if she's sexually active or experiences various symptoms, her healthcare provider may recommend a pelvic exam. Current ACOG recommendations don't indicate Pap tests for young women until they are at least twenty-one.

V-PROBLEMS YOU NEED TO KNOW ABOUT

Vulvas and vaginas can be affected by a number of health conditions; some of these produce noticeable symptoms and others do not. Although we've mentioned most of these conditions, we want to briefly highlight them here (for more detailed information about vulvovaginal health and medical conditions, we recommend checking out *The V Book* and, of course, speaking with your healthcare provider).[1]

Although yeast, or *candida albicans* (the scientific name for a common type of yeast), are normally found even in healthy vaginas, overgrowth of yeast can cause uncomfortable or even painful symptoms for women. As we mentioned earlier, if you suspect you have a **yeast infection**, we recommend checking in with a healthcare provider by telephone or in person for advice before treating yourself with over-the-counter medications, which can sometimes cause more harm than good.

Bacterial infections and imbalances of the vagina are common reasons why women visit their healthcare providers. Most are easily treatable. However, **bacterial vaginosis** (BV)—a condition in which the normal, healthy balance of the vagina is disrupted and certain bacteria seem to overgrow—is one condition that remains a challenge for many women, their partners, and their healthcare providers. Although some women who have BV are easily treated and never seem to experience a recurrence of their symptoms, other women have recurrent episodes of BV. Common symptoms of BV include itching, pain, burning, vaginal discharge, and genital odor (sometimes the odor is strongest after intercourse). According to the Centers for Disease Control and Prevention (CDC), BV is the most common vaginal infection among women who are of childbearing age.[16] Women who struggle with recurrent BV may be best helped by meeting with a vulvovaginal specialist who focuses on infections like BV (find one through issvd.org).

Genital warts are caused by certain strains of the human papillomavirus (HPV). They are usually small and painless. Some healthcare providers recommend a "wait and see" approach to genital warts, as they often do not cause discomfort and frequently go away on their own. Other times, treatment (which can include the use of a topical cream) is recommended. If you have been diagnosed with genital warts, ask your healthcare provider for his or her recommendation. As part of monthly vulvar self-examination, check on the status of your warts: if they increase in number or size, bring this to the attention of your healthcare provider. Don't be afraid to ask your healthcare provider for their thoughts on biopsying the warts to make sure they are indeed warts and not something else. Also, Gardasil (an HPV vaccine) protects against two strains that cause many cases of genital warts.

Genital herpes is caused by the herpes simplex virus and, like HPV, can be passed on during oral sex, vaginal sex, or anal sex. Genital herpes lesions can be very painful, perhaps particularly during the initial outbreak. Fortunately, antiviral medications are available that can reduce the frequency and severity of outbreaks.

Vulvodynia is a term that, according to the National Vulvodynia Association, refers to "chronic vulvar pain without an identifiable cause." Women may experience pain that's limited to the vulvar vestibule, which is the area around the vaginal opening. This type has been called **vulvar vestibulitis syndrome** or **localized or provoked vulvodynia**. A second type is called **generalized vulvodynia** and refers to pain at other parts of the vulva, such as the clitoris, labia, and/or vestibule. Women with vulvodynia may experience nearly constant pain or sporadic pain. Other conditions such as allergies, STIs, and genital skin disorders typically need to be ruled out before a diagnosis of vulvodynia is given. Unfortunately, women with vulvodynia often see a number of healthcare providers before receiving a diagnosis.

My experiences with vulvar vestibulitis have really influenced my feelings towards my genitals. I could either choose to be ashamed about this and feel bad about myself for not enjoying vaginal penetration, or I can accept that's how my genitals are and work with alternative forms of sexual expression while working on exercises to help me relax my vestibule muscles (such as biofeedback).

—ALANA, 22, Indiana

There are also a number of skin disorders that can affect a woman's genitals. One of these is a condition called **lichen sclerosus** (LS), which can affect women (and men) of all ages and can also affect nongenital skin. Women with LS often have white areas of skin on their genitals and may experience genital itching. With treatment (which often consists of topical creams), LS symptoms can often be managed. If a woman does not receive treatment, her vulvar skin may become more fragile and easily torn, and vaginal penetration and intercourse may become uncomfortable or painful.

Although not a v-problem per se, being **hypersensitive or allergic to semen** can certainly affect women's vulvas and vaginas (as well as have other health effects). If you experience genital irritation, burning, itching, or pain following unprotected intercourse with a man, or other forms of contact with his semen, try having sex with a condom the next time. If you don't have similar reactions, you might want to ask your healthcare provider about the possibility that you have a seminal allergy or sensitivity. Although rare, some women have severe allergic reactions to semen. Certainly, if you notice any health concerns during or after sex with a partner (such as difficulty swallowing or breathing, or breaking out in hives) seek emergency medical care. This is a relatively new area of research, so semen allergies are not well understood. Some women appear to be allergic to the semen of any man they have sex with; others seem to be allergic to the semen of only a particular man. Still, other women who have never experienced any reactions to men's semen suddenly develop sensitivities or allergies following a hormonal change, such as giving birth or going through menopause.

Finally, although rare, it is possible for women to develop cancer on their genitals. Early signs of **vulvar cancer** (spelled "vulval cancer" in the United Kingdom and Australia, among other countries) can include chronic itching as well as lumps or bumps on the genitals. This is challenging, as many non-cancerous conditions have similar symptoms. With early detection and treatment, vulvar cancer has a high survival rate. Performing vulvar self-examination can aid in the early detection of vulvar cancer and other conditions, such as **vulvar intraepithelial neoplasia** (VIN, considered a pre-cancerous condition of the vulva). Both vulvar cancer and VIN are linked to HPV. Cigarette smoking also appears to increase the risk of vulvar cancer and VIN. Although vulvar cancer and VIN used to be more often considered conditions of older women, an increasing number of young women have been diagnosed with vulvar cancer and VIN over the past decade.

INTERVIEW WITH KATH MAZZELLA, FOUNDER OF THE GYNAECOLOGICAL AWARENESS INFORMATION NETWORK

Can you tell us a bit about your background and how this work became so important to you?

With a strong family history of cancer, I had an abnormal Pap smear at the age of thirty-nine and eighteen months later, a lump appeared next to my clitoris. Over two years, I consulted two general practitioners and two gynaecologists who said it was common to have lumps in the vulva. I requested for the lump to be removed, which when biopsied was indeed cancer, and the removal of my clitoris, vulva, and lymph glands immediately followed. I was completely unprepared for what I faced personally and in society. The sadness was (is) so indescribable. Women in general are so unsuspecting and uninformed. I felt I had died as a woman and was now just an "it." In general, I discovered there was a shroud of secrecy and a willingness to suffer in silence with women. In my search for answers, I found the word pudendum (Latin, meaning *female genitalia; one who should and ought to be ashamed; the shameful part of a woman*). Then I noticed women were being taught that the vulva was a vagina and still most think this is so, keeping the pudendum mindset alive. Most viewed the vulva as pornographic and not as an incredible part of our anatomy. What does this say about women when we don't call our genitalia the correct terminology?

How did you form GAIN?

I met two other women who had radical vulvectomies, and being so isolated, mostly from women in a world that did not speak about "down there" or anything "gynae," I placed an advertisement in a woman's magazine. The replies of the women who wanted to pour their hearts out after years and years of suppression and suffering moved me, and I decided I had to find a way to stop this suppression. I noticed the advice being given was mostly from men—I saw a quote by a male gynaecologist—"What women won't talk about." I gathered my mother, my sisters, and my friends to help me work out how to form a support group for those too anxious to speak up after enduring such devastation.

Which GAIN/IGAD-related accomplishments are you most proud of and why?

1. After being treated like I was a crazy woman for speaking out as I did, the global letters of support for my vision for an International GYN Awareness Day is one of my greatest accomplishments.
2. Gaining Australian of the Year Professor Ian Frazer as GAIN Patron.
3. Giving voice to a woman who had her clitoris and vulva removed by a deranged gynecologist—getting the media involved and seeing legislation changed to offer more protection.
4. That I stood my own ground and didn't take no for an answer, and the empowerment I felt so that others can do the same.
5. Recipient of six awards, including the Order of Australia.

What do you wish more women knew about their vulval health?

I wish women could be more accepting that the vulva is a very important part of the body where life begins and it is so very, very precious. The more they understand about the vulva, the more empowering, for confidence lies within this knowledge.

What can women do to help raise awareness in their own communities?

As the vulva is still in the background of women's health, women could assist in their own communities by celebrating the International GYN Awareness Day—September 10—annually and making it fun and informative would give a good platform to raising a positive aspect to vulval health. All they have to do is to draw together medical practitioners and people from the community, invite a guest speaker to speak on a GYN-related topic, and sit around the table together and talk about it.

Men need the support just as much as the women. By inviting people to speak openly, we are allowing them the opportunity to receive the support they need, and it empowers everyone. Also by breaking down those barriers between medical professionals and their patients, a greater quality of care and treatment can be gained which benefits everyone.

For more information about Kath and her very important work, please check out Gynaecological Awareness Information Network (GAIN), Inc. (www.gain.org.au and www.kathmazzella.com).

OPENING UP: VAGINAL DILATORS

Vaginal dilators are sometimes described as "medical dildos." They often come in sets of five or six with the smallest being about the size of an adult's pinky finger and the largest being longer and thicker than an average-sized penis. Dilators may be used by women who have experienced vaginal narrowing or pain as a result of side effects from cancer treatments (such as pelvic radiation). They are also sometimes used as part of a larger treatment plan for women with vaginismus, vulvodynia, or other vulvovaginal pain conditions. In addition, some women who have very small vaginas—as is sometimes the case with women who have a condition called androgen insensitivity syndrome (AIS)—find that using dilators can help them stretch their vaginas. Surgeons may also suggest that their patients who have male-to-female sex-reassignment surgery use dilators to help stretch their "neo-vagina" (the surgically created vagina).

Dilators can be purchased online or through some healthcare providers and sex therapists. Some women use dilators in order to overcome a pain disorder that keeps them from having sex with a partner. Others use a dilator to prevent sexual-function problems or to treat sexual side effects. Still, these are not the only reasons why dilator use can be helpful or important.

As mentioned, some cancer treatments can result in a woman's vagina narrowing substantially. Not only can this make sexual intercourse feel difficult, if not impossible, but it can also make it very difficult for a healthcare provider to properly examine a woman's vagina and cervix during a GYN exam. This is particularly important as healthcare providers will want to be able to properly view and examine the cervix so that they can make sure that a woman does not develop or have a recurrence of cervical cancer, among other issues. Dilator therapy can help women maintain their vaginal patency (a fancy term that basically means vaginal flexibility and tone, allowing it to open enough to be viewed during exams).

How It Works

Dilators can be used in many different ways. Women who use them as part of a treatment plan recommended by a healthcare provider or sex therapist should ask their provider/therapist for specific recommendations. Generally speaking, women are advised to begin with the smallest dilator and partially insert it into their vagina, often with water-based lubricant applied to the dilator to ease penetration. Women may move it in and out if they want, but often, they will just leave it there for ten minutes or longer so that the vagina gets used to accommodating an object of that size. As that size becomes more comfortable, women may be advised to move to the next size and repeat the cycle until she has gotten to the size that she, in consultation with her healthcare provider, has decided she wants to use. For some women, the process of moving through the dilator sizes takes weeks. For others, it takes months. Similarly, some women insert the dilator while lying down and reading or watching television, while other women make dilator use a part of masturbation or sex play with a partner. There are many different ways that women experience dilator use. See the Resources section for shops that may carry dilators.

YOUR HEALTHY HOOHA

Although there are many things that can go wrong with the vulva and vagina, there are also many things that can go right. Every day, you have opportunities to care for your genital parts—to wash them carefully, to wear clothes that let them breathe, to choose partners and doctors that take care of them, and to love them so much that you take the time to check them out every now and then just to make sure they're all right. This is the best that we can ask of ourselves. And if something does go wrong, we hope that the information in this chapter helps you figure out how to get the help and, if relevant, the treatment that you need. Here's to looking forward to a world of healthy vulvas and vaginas!

TEST YOUR VQ

1. Pantyliners are best used
   a. every day
   b. whenever vaginal discharge is present
   c. only when a woman is menstruating
   d. all of the above

2. Aside from yeast infections, vaginal itching may be caused by
   a. ingredients in lubricants
   b. bath products
   c. wearing tight, restrictive clothing that traps moisture
   d. all of the above

3. Current recommendations are for young women to have their first gynecological exam
   a. by age twelve
   b. between the ages of thirteen and fifteen
   c. at age eighteen
   d. at age twenty-one

Answers

1. c
2. d
3. b

· 3 ·

Vulvalicious

Vulvas and Vaginas in Bed

$\mathscr{I}$n spite of the significant efforts and good intentions of highly dedicated genital admirers, the vulva and vagina remain a mystery for
many—especially when it comes to sex and pleasure. In some ways,
this is not terribly shocking, given that women's bodies and sexual
response are not fully understood even by scientists and medical doctors. In other ways, it's quite sad to not be able to unlock the pleasures
of parts we live with on a daily basis.

Unfortunately, a lack of knowledge about women's bodies and
sexuality can pose challenges for people's sexual lives. Women may
feel frustrated if they don't know how they like to be touched on
their genitals or where they liked to be touched. They may feel
guilty or embarrassed about masturbating, even though most women
masturbate.[1] Also, many men and women who have sex with women
feel equally mystified about women's bodies. They may not be sure
how to touch or lick their girlfriend or wife in order to please her
sexually.

It's really weird living with genitals I don't like the look of in general. I like
the feeling of intercourse/masturbation, but when I am with a woman, I feel
bad that I don't want to reciprocate anything. I'm also scared that after seeing
me give birth, my husband's not going to want to go down there.

—LILLY, 23, California

83

In the first chapter, we took an introductory look at the parts of the vulva and vagina. We learned, for example, that the clitoris is an incredibly nerve-rich part of a woman's body, packed with about eight thousand nerve endings in a pretty small space. Yet, as fabulous as the clitoris's potential role during sex may be, it's certainly not the only part of the vulva or vagina that's relevant to sex or sensual pleasure. Each and every part of women's genitals has some level of erotic potential or role to play in sexual play or sexual response.

In this chapter, we will provide you with information about the vulva, vagina, and sex—including a few tips related to sex toys—so that you can feel confident in and out of bed, whether you're pleasuring yourself or showing your partner what you find most enjoyable or erotic.

THE AGE OF CLIT-ARIUS

The clitoris is highly sensitive thanks to all the nerve endings inside of it, but there's more to it than nerves. The clitoris was first scientifically detailed in its full size and glory in 1998,[2] which means that the scientific study of the clitoris is actually quite young.

I wish more women would think beyond the clitoris. We make jokes about men who can't find it or similar when, really, the whole area is so sensitive. We are missing out if we just encourage our partners to go for the high point every time, not to mention risking pain thinking the glans is all she wrote.

—JEAN, 32, New Mexico

Sure, we knew about the clitoris long before 1998, but—outside of progressive feminist health books and medical circles—it was more commonly thought of as a little nubby thing that was small and mostly on the outside of the body. Following on the heels of earlier work, Dr. Helen O'Connell's team[2] published anatomical evidence that showed that the clitoris is much larger than meets the eye and that it is made up of a variety of parts, like the crura (which are two branches that extend backward into the body and swell during sexual arousal) and the bulbs of the clitoris.[2] This got people thinking about the clitoris and about women's sexuality more generally. The size and placement of the clitoris means that the clitoris can be stimulated from various types of touch. One can stimulate the glans clitoris (the part one can see from the outside) with fingers or a vibrator during masturbation alone or with a partner. The glans clitoris can also be stimulated with a tongue, lips, or fingers during cunnilingus, as it often responds to light touch. Also, the inside parts of the clitoris can be indirectly stimulated during vaginal penetration with fingers, a partner's penis, or a sex toy such as a dildo or vibrator. Because some clitoral parts are deeper inside the body, firm pressure may be a better option for internal stimulation of the clitoris.

I never liked any part of being a woman, especially my genitals, until I was 19 and in my second year of college. After seeing The Vagina Monologues *and breaking away from my home town and family's negative view of women and their sexuality, I began to look into these things for myself. I unfortunately did not begin masturbating until I was 19, and finally had sexual experiences when I was 20. Since I am only interested and attracted to women, I had a somewhat good and helpful idea of what to do during my first sexual experiences since as a woman, I know what women might generally like.*

—DAWN, 20, Ohio

As such, vaginal penetration can deliver both vaginal stimulation as well as stimulation of the inside branches of the clitoris (the crura)—and, if you remember from chapter 1—it's this indirect way of stimulating the clitoris through the vaginal walls that may be what's at the heart of the G-spot. After all, when a woman becomes sexually excited and aroused, blood flows to her pelvic area and genitals. The clitoris becomes enlarged during this process, which can make the area more easily stimulated and more sensitive to stimulation.

The clitoris isn't the only part to change in response to sexy times. More recently, Dr. O'Connell—after further study of the clitoris and women's genital parts—came to another conclusion. She noted that the clitoris doesn't seem to function in a vacuum. Rather, she suggested we consider using the term "clitoral complex" to describe the unique interplay among the clitoris, vagina, and urethra.[3] If one of these parts is moved, then the other parts move and are thus stimulated as well, though not in a uniform way. Let's take penile-vaginal intercourse as an example. When a man's penis and a woman's vagina are in intercourse, her vagina expands to accommodate his penis. Thus, the vagina is affected—it gets bigger and is stimulated on all of its walls. But the inside parts of the clitoris are likely stimulated, too, and the urethra is pushed a bit upward, as well. This is an important way of thinking about women's bodies because it takes us away from a simplistic model of sex, in which only the vagina is stimulated during intercourse, to a more complex way of thinking about sex, in which the vagina, urethra, and clitoris are all stimulated and impacted during intercourse.

I wish that more women knew that for a lot of women, vaginal intercourse is NOT the most satisfying sexual activity and therefore there is NOTHING wrong with women who do not "get off" on vaginal intercourse. I think this would increase the quality of women's sex lives as they're able to explore alternative options (such as anal intercourse, oral sex, vibrators, etc.).

—ALANA, 22, Indiana

THE EXCITED VULVA AND VAGINA

During sexual excitement, increased blood flow to the genital area means changes for the entire genital area. The labia minora (inner lips) are filled with blood vessels. This means that during sexual arousal, when these blood vessels engorge with blood, the labia may appear larger than usual. With increased blood flow, they may also develop into a deeper shade of pink, red, or purple. Some scientists believe that the mons pubis (the triangular area where hair often grows; also called the "mons") is a site where pheromones are released and that pubic hair may trap pheromones that can be "read" by potential partners as a sort of sexual signal.[4] Still, it's not known whether pubic hair truly serves this pheromone-trapping function or not.

Some people also feel that sexual arousal and excitement change how the G-spot area of the vagina feels, with some saying that the G-spot feels harder or more pronounced when a woman is sexually excited. If you're curious about trying G-spot stimulation, you may want to try first arousing yourself through fantasy, dirty talk, clitoral stimulation, kissing, watching porn, touching your partner (and being touched), or whatever else turns you on. Once you feel sufficiently excited or aroused, you may find it easier to locate your own G-spot. If you're interested in engaging in a little G-spot exploration with a female partner, try building her arousal through breast play, kissing, or whatever gets her motor humming for at least ten or fifteen minutes before attempting G-spot stimulation. It may be that her G-spot is easier for you or her to find—or at the very least that her G-spot exploration is more comfortable—once the vagina has had more of a chance to lubricate during arousal.

TRANSUDATE: A BORING WORD WITH EXCITING IMPLICATIONS

Speaking of vaginal lubrication, did you know that sexual excitement is one of the leading triggers for vaginal wetness and natural lubrication? Here's how: as blood flows to the genitals during sexual excitement and arousal, something cool happens. Transudate (basically, a clear part of the blood) passes through the blood vessels and vaginal walls, where it lubricates the walls and thus gets the name "vaginal lubrication" or, more casually, "vaginal wetness."[5] This is one reason why sexual excitement and arousal are key to vaginal lubrication. If a woman and her partner skip foreplay or don't spend

MEN TALK MUFFS

We asked men what they like about women's genitals and whether there are certain qualities that they prefer over others. Here's what they had to say:

"Moisture, warmth."—Andres, 31, Spain

"I have only ever been with my girlfriend, so I have no base of comparison, but I can definitely say that I like to feel how soft and warm her genitals are. I like how slick she gets when I excite her and her heady scent. I like her hair, how it collects her pheromones and the rush I get when I pleasure her orally. Sometimes I get a hair on the back of my tongue but that's nothing to harp about in comparison to stroking her soft hair and her labia while we wind down after making love."—Chris, 22, Canada

"I like a little pubic hair verses a vagina being shaved bare."—John, 36, Georgia

"Taste, smell, less hair is better, lubricated."—Austin, 31, Wisconsin

"Large clit, large lips (labia)."—Peter, 46, Illinois

"I think there is something inherently magical about seeing a woman's vagina glistening."—Tyrese, 25, Virginia

"I like the soft feel, the folds to explore, the way they can get me excited."—Dan, 51, Massachusetts

"Everything! The variety of shapes and colours. The hair. I much prefer genitals with hair. I also like exposed/protruding inner labia. I just think female genitals are hugely interesting and attractive—much more than people generally think."—Henry, 60, UK

"Love the shape of them and how each one is different from the other. Also like the metallic taste when it is soft (not too strong). Nice smell and overall cleanliness is also something that I really like. I also like the complexity of the vagina, especially when compared to the penis. It is much more intricate and varied, and it is great to learn how every woman gets pleasure from her vagina in a slightly (or completely different) way."—Victor, 30, Peru

"They look like a flower. Like an orchid. I like them best when they have some exterior vulva. Like, after a woman has had a child, they are sexier looking. I like them shaved so that nothing covers the view of them. I like the scent and taste. I love it when some of the skin pulls outward and pushes inward on each stroke. I like how they are so close to the woman's anus. One good lick can hit both spots. I love it when they trickle liquid from a woman's excitement. I love how the inside of their pussy feels when I insert a finger or two. I love to find and rub the G-spot while licking them."—Tom, 45, New York

"The heat, the slickness, tightness, the structure of the labia appeals to me, and the aesthetics and feel of the clitoris are also great. The parts I feel are more important than the parts I see."—Patrick, 18, Canada

"I prefer hairy, but not on the thighs. I prefer long inner lips. I prefer darker color. I prefer large clitoris and hood."—Ben, 70, Canada

"I like how dynamic they are, depending on the state of arousal. I like how they feel when they are wet from excitement. I like how they taste, look and smell. I love the clitoris."—Mike, 44, Taiwan

"It is like a mystery cave over the years I have figured out spots that are good hiding areas and can arouse a woman."—Klaus, 32, New York

"Bald, smells nice. Tastes delicious. When it squirts, it's nice."—Mark, 31, Canada

"They look so beautiful, and they feel so beautiful. They have lovely variations in texture, changing with increasing wetness. The way in which the vulva opens up with increasing excitement is as welcoming as anything humanly possible. The delicately shifting folds, the kissable accessible bits, the lickable less-accessible bits, the let's-feel-how-deep-this-goes remoter bits—they're all delectable. Pubic hair—lovely stuff—good to stroke, to tease, to feel scratching my belly."—William, 48, UK

"I like the softness of the area in general, how easily it responds to a touch. I like how it is always warm. I don't have a preference for pronounced or minimal inner or outer labial areas that I'm aware of. I like the general shape and how the lines of the body seem to converge there. I usually like the taste and smells associated with a woman's genitals."—Joe, 29, Georgia

"The softness, when it is wet, the way it expands and conforms to the shape of my penis."—Don, 49, Missouri

"They are a beautiful, complex creation. They turn me on, particularly my partner's. I like that she has very little hair near her outer lips (naturally) but hair on her mons. This makes oral sex very enjoyable for me, but also gives her a 'womanly' look."—Stephen, 28, Minnesota

"They are a welcoming place of total love. They say, cum and stay a while, as you are, completely and wholly accepted."—Brian, 45, Minnesota

"I like long, smooth, symmetrical lips—something voluptuous that captures the gaze and imagination. I like large clits, but I don't get as excited over them as I do over lips and hoods. I like a vulva to be big, lips unfurled, and deep in its cleft. And scent is very important—some scents are profoundly more attractive than others. And wetness—I like her to produce as much come as possible, whether watery or thick. I love cunts :)"—Adam, 31, Maine

"Taste, smell, feel. I like pubic hair, so I prefer it when women do not remove all of it."—Gary, 23, Oklahoma

time on arousal and just jump into sex, then there may not be enough time for blood to flow to the genitals in any significant amount. If blood flow doesn't increase to the genitals, then the transudation process isn't going to happen. And if transudation doesn't occur, then there's not going to be much vaginal lubrication to make penetration more slippery, comfortable, and pleasurable.

Mostly, I only enjoy clitoral stimulation because penetration is not that enjoyable unless it's a really big penis. I don't seem to feel anything in the first few inches, which I have always found strange.

—CLARA, 21, Ireland

That said, excitement isn't the only key to unlocking the door to the castle of vaginal lubrication. A woman's estrogen levels are also important to vaginal lubrication.[5] Even young babies (who have high levels of estrogen thanks to having just come from their mom's body) experience vaginal lubrication.[6] As girls go through puberty and experience increases in estrogen, they again may notice extra amounts of vaginal wetness even when they don't feel aroused or excited. This is, in part, why women may notice changes in their natural vaginal wetness throughout their menstrual cycle, as estrogen levels change during their cycle. When estrogen levels are low—such as when a woman is breastfeeding or when she approaches menopause or is postmenopausal—she may experience vaginal dryness. Women who take low-dose estrogen birth-control pills may also notice less vaginal lubrication. The bottom line is that estrogen plays a big role in vaginal lubrication and wetness. If you ever notice significant changes to your experience of vaginal lubrication even though you're feeling sexually aroused, it's worth asking your healthcare provider to look further into the issue, as your hormones may be partially responsible.

LOW TIDE

Although people often associate vaginal dryness and lubrication difficulties with menopause, women of all ages may experience related problems from time to time. In our recent study, the National Survey of Sexual Health and Behavior (NSSHB), we found that nearly one-third of women ages eighteen to fifty-nine experienced difficulties with lubrication during their most recent sexual encounter.[7] Specifically, vaginal lubrication difficulties during the most recent sexual event were reported by

- 35.1 percent of women ages 18–24
- 29.1 percent of women ages 25–29
- 31.5 percent of women ages 30–39

- 36.1 percent of women ages 40–49
- 48.3 percent of women ages 50–59
- 65.2 percent of women ages 60–69

That's a lot of women reporting difficulty with vaginal lubrication! And as you can see, although vaginal-lubrication problems are more common among older women, it's not only a problem for older women. Even many young women—35 percent of college-aged women—experience such difficulties on occasion. Because young women's bodies should be able to produce natural vaginal lubrication on their own, we're guessing that many of these women's sexual experiences could be improved by relaxing and spending more time in foreplay or exciting sex play prior to penetration.

I've experienced all kinds of orgasms, double orgasms, cascade orgasms that lasted for minutes, all kinds. But I think my favorite happened when I was stuck in rush hour traffic in a major midwest city. It was bumper to bumper, and was late in the year, so it was dark already. I was bored, so I got a wild idea and got my vibrator out of my bag (I was driving home from a weekend away). And I masturbated while I inched along the expressway. When I came, I yelled so loudly, I wondered if other people in other cars could hear me. That was part of the thrill; I was in public, doing something forbidden, and it was fantastic.

—KELLY, 25, Illinois

Lubrication helps to decrease friction and, in turn, can help sex to feel more comfortable and pleasurable. It can also reduce the risk of a woman experiencing vaginal cuts and tears during vaginal penetration or intercourse. Vaginal dryness, on the other hand, can make sex feel tight (in a not-very-pleasant way for most) and may be uncomfortable for both partners. As such, it may be worth your time to learn how to enhance your natural vaginal lubrication—or call in the reinforcements (store-bought lube) when wanted or needed.

WAYS TO GET WET

What can you do to have more pleasurable, comfortable sex? Here are a few ideas:

1. **Spend more time in foreplay (or whatever it is that feels exciting to you and your partner).** This will allow your body to have sufficient time to "warm up," meaning more time for blood flow to increase to the genitals, for transudation to happen, and consequently, for natural lubrication to kick in. Aim for spending at least ten or fifteen minutes doing something that feels arousing for you. It might be breast play, sex-toy play, oral sex, massage, dirty talk, or reading or watching erotica together that turns you on. When you and your body feel ready to romp (a feeling of vaginal throbbing is often a good sign!), chances are that your vagina will be ready, too, with sufficient wetness.

2. **Create optimal conditions for sex.** If you like to shower or take a bath before sex, wait to have sex until you've relaxed for a while post-shower/bath. Why? Because taking a bath or shower can dry the vagina—just as it turns the rest of our skin into wrinkly "prunes" after a long bath or swim. Taking time to let the vaginal tissues re-hydrate can help.

3. **Talk to your healthcare provider.** It may be that your vaginal-lubrication difficulties are related to medications, aging, breastfeeding, or medical conditions that you may be experiencing.

4. **Choose wisely.** If you and a sexual partner are using condoms, choose lubricated condoms. They can help to decrease friction and make sex feel more comfortable.

5. **Ask your healthcare provider about a vaginal moisturizer.** If you are experiencing ongoing issues with vaginal dryness, then a vaginal moisturizer might be right for you. Some

moisturizers are enhanced with hormones, and others do not contain hormones. If you have a history of breast cancer or are otherwise concerned about hormones, let your healthcare provider know. Vaginal moisturizers are often applied at night before bed by using an applicator that delivers moisture to the vagina. Using a vaginal moisturizer often leaves the vagina feeling moist for several days.

6. **Consider using a lubricant.** Water-based lubricants and silicone-based lubricants can be used with latex condoms. Steer clear of oil-based lubricants if you're using latex condoms, as they can cause latex condoms to break. If you're using silicone sex toys or birth control (such as a silicone diaphragm or cervical cap), choose a water-based lubricant over a silicone-based lubricant, as the latter may degrade or damage silicone products. Research that we've conducted at the Center for Sexual Health Promotion and published in 2011 in the *Journal of Sexual Medicine* shows that when women used the water-based or silicone-based lubricants in our study, they generally rated sex as more pleasurable and satisfying than when they didn't use lubricant.[8] That said, other researchers have found that some lubricants may slow down sperm and thus may not be good choices for people trying to become pregnant. If you're trying to conceive, ask your healthcare provider for his or her opinion about Pre-Seed or other lubricants that have been designed to be more friendly to sperm.

WHAT YOUR V-PARTS HAVE TO DO WITH THE BIG O

You've probably read about different "types" of orgasm. Perhaps you have personally felt that your orgasms feel different depending on the type of stimulation. Or maybe you've never had an orgasm, or have experienced them only rarely, but you've heard about orgasm types and have been curious about them. Often people divide orgasms into the categories of vaginal orgasm, clitoral orgasm, uterine orgasm, and blended orgasm, though some people use different terms or add on additional categories.[9]

Findings from scientific research suggest that the clitoris is likely involved in most if not all of women's orgasms—even if the glans clitoris itself isn't directly stimulated.[9] Remember that "clitoral complex" and how vaginal penetration can stimulate the clitoris, too? That just goes to show you how complicated this can get very quickly. What may look like one type of orgasm (for example, an orgasm from vaginal intercourse) may be an orgasm that involves the clitoris—not just the vagina. So is that a vaginal orgasm, a clitoral orgasm, a G-spot orgasm (if it was stimulation of that one part of the vagina that pushed a woman over her orgasmic edge), or something else? Good question—we don't know! Scientists are still trying to understand the female orgasm including the many ways that people try to categorize it.

What we *do* know is that there are various nerve pathways linked to orgasm. In women, there are at least four nerve pathways that convey sensory information from certain genital and reproductive organs to the brain. The **pudendal nerve** conveys sensory information from the clitoris to the brain, so this is the pathway for clitoral stimulation that may result in an orgasm. The **pelvic nerve** conveys sensory information from a woman's cervix and vagina up to her brain, whereas the **hypogastric nerve** serves the uterus and cervix. More recently identified as part of sexual response is the **vagus nerve**, which carries sensory information from the cervix and uterus to the brain, bypassing the spinal cord. (For more information about each of these nerve pathways, check out Komisaruk, Beyer-Flores, and Whipple's 2006 book, *The Science of Orgasm*.[10])

I wish there was more information out there to counteract the porno view that women can have orgasms—instantly—from vaginal penetration. It annoys me to no end that some women think they're ill if they can't do this, and a lot of guys seem to believe it to be the case as well.

—JEN, 23, Canada

V-CRAFT: PLEASURE PANTIES

Perhaps you've seen reflexology socks or gloves? They are socks or gloves that are adorned with a "map" of the various pressure points and other points of stimulation so that a person can wear them and either stimulate their own feet or hands or have a friend or partner do it for them, according to the map.

Years ago, when Debby was first acting in *The Vagina Monologues* and getting into vulva and vagina art, she came up with an idea for DIY vulva panties—also called "pleasure panties." Here's how you can make your own.

What You Will Need

- 1 pair of white or lightly colored cotton underwear (full or partial bottom, not a thong or G-string)
- permanent markers in different colors (the kind that you can use to draw on clothing that won't bleed or wash off in the laundry)
- a friend or partner (helpful but not necessary)

What to Do

While wearing the underwear, ask your partner to help you outline the parts of your vulva on the side of the panties facing him or her. Your friend/partner might draw a circle or oval where your glans clitoris is. Your inner and outer labia can also be traced. Remember, too, to include your mons, vaginal entrance, perineum, and, if you so desire, your anal opening, too (it can be a little tricky to get all the way there for some, but spreading one's legs can make for easier access).

You might want to ask your partner to use different colors for various parts. You can then take your panties off and use the outline

Knowing about these nerve pathways may help you to understand how women can have a wide range of experiences related to orgasm. Vaginal intercourse may end up stimulating the vagina as well as the clitoris and cervix, which may mean that any of the previously

to write words on the panties. You can be precise, if you want, and label the parts of your vulva and anus (e.g., "clitoris," etc.). Or, instead, you can write how you like to be touched—for example, you can write, "Softly here," or "More attention here, please!" Alternatively, you can use design schemes, such as a red "X" to mark the spot(s) where you like to be touched (or the parts to avoid touching directly).

Some Tips

- Some markers may ink through the panties, meaning you may end up getting ink on your vulva. Some women don't mind this. Others—particularly those with sensitive skin—might wish to avoid this. To reduce the likelihood of inking through to your genital parts, wear two or three layers of underwear while you make your pleasure panties. Although collaborating with a partner can make this easier, having a friend or partner on hand is not necessary; you can make pleasure panties by yourself. Wearing them and looking in a mirror at the same time can be helpful.
- Have fun! Be creative about what you want to map out. Perhaps you'd like to map out the order of how you'd like to be touched, such as writing a number one on the first place you'd like your partner to touch you before proceeding to the part labeled two.
- Making pleasure panties with a partner can be a great way to spruce up your sex life. It creates space for you to talk about your vulva parts and what kind of stimulation you do or don't like. In turn, it creates opportunities for your partner to learn about your preferences for touching, licking, and various types of sex play. It can also be a very sexy way to initiate foreplay and to add a playful—dare we say, crafty—dimension to sex.

listed nerve pathways—and maybe others, too—carry information to the brain in a way that results in orgasm. While not all women experience orgasm, the vast majority of women are capable of experiencing orgasm, though it may take time, patience, and practice to do so. Also, not all women want to experience orgasm (perhaps especially if they are prone to orgasm-related migraines or other painful experiences) or care to, even if they've had them before and enjoyed them. But for those who do want to experience orgasm, this growing area of research may be helpful.

We don't fully understand how orgasms occur—specifically, how a woman goes from Point A (some type of sexual stimulation) to Point B (experiencing an orgasm), although this is an area that scientists are trying to better understand. What we do know is that, although the exact process of female orgasm is yet to be discovered, we don't have to wait for science to catch up in order to experience the joys of sexual pleasure and/or orgasm.

PARTNERED PLAY TO PLEASURE YOUR POONANNY

For all of the heartbreak and loss of human lives associated with the ongoing HIV epidemic, a positive change to come out of this period of the 1980s is that healthcare providers, public-health professionals, and sex and health educators began talking more openly about safer—but still pleasurable—sex. By expanding conversations about "sex" to include more than just vaginal or anal sex, sexual health professionals have hoped to introduce men and women to a range of ways in which people can pleasure each other while reducing the risk of spreading infections, such as HIV. Ultimately, safer-sex messages are about saving lives.

Partnered masturbation is one of the safest forms of sex between two or more people. It's also a type of sex that many people are familiar with, if for no other reason than that it's similar to how a lot of teenagers and young adults start out relating sexually with each other—touching each other's genitals (through fingering and/or hand jobs), sometimes to the point of orgasm and other times not.

ACTIVITY: MASTER YOUR MASTURBATION

The vast majority of women masturbate—according to the NSSHB, more than 80 percent of women in their twenties and thirties have masturbated[1]—but just how women masturbate can vary not only from woman to woman but also from day to day. How you enjoy masturbation tonight may be very different than what you feel like doing next week or next year. As with partnered sex, it sometimes pays to vary your masturbation rather than stick with the same old, boring routine. Here are some ideas for setting the scene for pleasurable masturbation:

- Light candles to set a sensual mood for pleasure.
- Watch your favorite porn, such as a DVD that you own or have rented, or an online video.
- Lay a soft blanket on the floor, perhaps in front of a fireplace (if you have one) or candles, and lay down or kneel on the blanket for your masturbation (for safety, keep a safe distance from the fireplace or candles).
- Put fresh sheets on the bed and christen it with a self-pleasuring session.
- Use a vibrator to massage other body parts, such as your back, thighs, or breasts, before using it to stimulate your own genitals.
- Position yourself in front of a mirror.
- Take a waterproof sex toy into the bath or shower for a steamy private-sex session.

You might also explore your inside parts (the vagina) as well as your outside parts (the clitoris, labia, etc.). Watching in a mirror as you stimulate your vulva and/or vagina can be sexy, too.

Know your own style for setting the mood, as well as for how you like to stimulate yourself—but do try to be brave about exploring. Sometimes particularly delicious pleasures lie in trying something new.

People can't get pregnant from touching each other's genitals—assuming, of course, that a woman doesn't let a male partner ejaculate on her hand and then insert her semen-covered finger near or in her vaginal opening (or engage in some other behavior that would result in semen getting close to or in the vagina). It is also unlikely that people will pass STIs to one another through partnered masturbation, which makes it a much safer form of sexual expression than vaginal or anal sex.

There are many ways to enhance the quality of partnered masturbation. Here, we'll focus on ways to use various body parts—except for the lips, tongue, mouth, or penis (which we'll tackle soon enough)—to stimulate a woman's vagina and/or vulva during partnered play.

- **Ask for a tug.** The mons pubis is a sensitive area for many women. In the same way that many women enjoy having a partner run their fingers through the hair on their heads, a woman may also enjoy having a partner sensually run his/her fingers through or gently tug on her pubic hair. This can be a sensuous prelude or complement to partnered masturbation. For some women, this can be an incredible way to build arousal during foreplay or sex play.
- **Vulva massage.** There are many ways to use one's hand to pleasure a woman's vulva. Ask your partner to use the heel of the palm of his/her hand to gently apply pressure to the mons or outer edges of the outer labia. You might also find it pleasurable if your partner gently uses his/her fingers to trace your vulva parts. If you enjoy vaginal penetration, then once sufficient arousal and lubrication have been built up, you may be turned on by having your partner insert a finger or two into your vagina while they gently massage the front, back, and/or side walls of your vagina.

A sex partner who loves your vulva is a wonderful, validating experience—I wish it for every woman.

—EMMA, 63, Oregon

- **Like to lap dance?** Try using your vulva to stimulate your partner—and simultaneously, yourself, too. Women may be stimulated by rubbing their vulvas against a man's erect penis or her female partner's vulva—even if their partner is wearing clothes. Even when both people are clothed, a woman can sometimes feel the contours of her partner's genitals via the movements of her thighs and vulva. And even when heavy clothes don't allow for a woman to feel everything she wants to, the warmth between both bodies, and the excitement of sitting on a partner's lap, kissing one another, or grinding, can be enormously arousing.
- **One finger at a time.** Gentle pressure on the front wall of a woman's vagina has been shown to increase a woman's threshold for pain (meaning that there's something about front-wall stimulation that may close a woman off to low-levels of pain and open her to more possibilities of pleasure). Wait until you are well lubricated, naturally or by way of a store-bought lubricant on your genitals and/or your partner's fingers. Ask your partner to slip one finger inside your vagina, gently but firmly sliding against the front wall. If or when you're ready for more, gradually ask him or her to increase stimulation one finger at a time.
- **Play footsies.** The foot is an often-underutilized sex toy. While lying down, legs apart, have your partner sit apart from you on a bed, or ask your partner to stand above you. Then, have your partner gently use his/her toes (make sure they're clean with trimmed toenails first) to stimulate your inner thigh and the parts of your vulva. Some women even like for

their partner to dip their big toe inside their vagina. Unconventional? Yes. But also, perhaps, unexpectedly fun.

- **Take charge.** While your partner is lying down, get on top cowgirl style, then lean back, resting on your forearms and elbows. From this position, you can use your vulva to stimulate your partner's penis or strap-on, by sliding your vulva up and down the shaft.
- **Dry hump each other**. Also called outercourse, dry humping can be a highly pleasurable way of stimulating each other's genitals without hands, tongues, or sex toys. All it takes is two people rolling around naked, clothed, or wearing only underwear, and having an awful lot of fun rubbing each other's bodies, high-school style.

SMOOCHIE COOCHIE: THE YUMMY WORLD OF CUNNILINGUS

Some women find it easier to experience orgasm while receiving cunnilingus than during other types of sex, such as vaginal intercourse. Even for women who don't experience orgasm from cunnilingus, receiving oral sex can be a pleasurable experience—a chance to sit or lie back and be attended to by one's partner. That's not to say that cunnilingus is always a passive, sit-back-let-go-and-be-worshipped experience. Cunnilingus can be an extremely active and take-charge experience for the woman on the receiving end. Here are several ways to tweak cunnilingus for maximum vulva and vagina pleasure:

- **The Ice Cream Trick.** Dreaded by some, longed for by others, this involves having your partner lick your vulva as if it were an ice cream cone: think long, savory, delicious licks of wonder.
- **Lick a message to your partner.** Perhaps you've played the massage game in which one person uses his/her finger to

"write" a message on a friend's back so that the friend has to guess what he/she is writing. This is similar, except it involves the vulva. Some people make it into a game, with the woman receiving cunnilingus having to guess the message. Other cunnilinguists don't tell their partners what they're up to; they simply find that spelling out a message like "I love you" or "You're hot" or "Vulvas are the best thing ever ever ever" (over and over again) can be an enjoyable way to concentrate on what they're doing.

SAY NO TO BLOW!

You may have heard about the dangers of blowing air into the vagina during oral sex, for fear of causing an air embolism (basically, air that doesn't belong in the cardiovascular system). Although it would be very rare to cause an air embolism by blowing air into the vagina, it is a possible outcome (and a dangerous possibility) and thus, we do not recommend this practice. Instead, have your partner kiss, lick, or gently nibble your vulva parts—he or she can save the blowing for gently blowing warm air on your inner thighs, breasts, or neck.

- **Constant flicks.** Some women—perhaps particularly those who enjoy the consistent stimulation provided by vibrators—enjoy constant tongue flicking as part of oral sex. If you don't like it when your partner switches things up down there, ask for constant flicks. Your partner may be able to stay focused by breathing in and out, or counting flicks. Keep a glass of water nearby for your partner if you desire or require lengthy stimulation for reasons of pleasure or orgasm. And if he or she tires out at first? No worries: it can take practice to build up endurance. The good news is that, while your partner is learning to build up endurance, you can switch to other types of sex play. Plus, practice can be a lot of fun—but everyone deserves a break.

- **Be kissed 'round the clock.** Starting at the twelve o'clock position (your glans clitoris), ask your partner to sprinkle kisses at each "numbered" position around your vulva as if it were a clock face. Or be kissed in a random pattern. For some women, kissing alone—albeit often prolonged kissing—is enough to drive them wild and/or bring them to orgasm.

- **To finger or not to finger?** Women have different preferences when it comes to fingers and oral sex. Some women find that it increases their arousal when their partner fingers them during oral sex. This may be especially true for those women who are responsive to vaginal-wall stimulation, such as G-spot stimulation. For other women, the added finger is a distraction that takes away from the general deliciousness of cunnilingus. You might explore both options to see what you like. You might also ask your partner what he or she thinks about the finger option. Oh, and make sure to be specific about where you want a finger, as some women would love to have a finger during cunnilingus but in their anus (not the vagina).

- **Two fingers?** There are also women who, at times, want a finger in both orifices, a la double penetration. This can be done with a well-lubricated thumb in one hole and a well-lubricated pointer finger in the other hole. Wearing a condom over one's finger is advisable for anal penetration, especially if you think you might switch to more vaginal play later on. It's better to avoid getting fecal matter in or near the vagina. Another option is to insert a condom-clad butt plug into the anus and/or a condom-clad dildo in the vagina while your partner does the whole mouth/tongue thing on the vulva.

- **Hold your partner's head**. It can feel very sexy for both partners to engage not just in a little hand holding, but in head holding as well. This doesn't have to feel like a domination/submission scene, unless that's your thing. Some people simply find it sexy to feel as though they are showing their partner what they like—or insisting on what they want (or being shown, as the case may be). Plus, it can be helpful to place a hand on your partner's head. When things are going well, you might press down more during excitement, thus giving your partner feedback about what's working so nicely for you and your vulva.

- **Sit on your partner's face.** Whether you're having oral sex in a bed, on a sofa, on the floor or in the backseat of a car, there is often room to sit on one's partner's face for oral sex. (In the backseat of a car, one can often press against the roof or hold on to the dry cleaning handles on the roof for more leverage.) If you ever get super into this type of sex, consider buying or making your own queening chair (a special chair or stool with a hole cut out in the middle so that a woman can sit on her lover's face for long periods of time while her partner performs oral sex on her; this is sometimes used as part of power-play activities).

I love looking at vaginas. Usually I look when I am about to go down on someone and seeing it fills me with such anticipation. I think I was too scared of my own sexuality to ever really look/compare with friends growing up.
—LINDSEY, 23, Washington

- **Side-by-side 69.** Side-by-side oral sex is sometimes thought of as a yin-yang, with both partners giving and receiving in perfect harmony. Oh, the romance of it all! Of course, it can be awkward for some to try to concentrate on giving when they're having so much fun receiving, but a challenge can be a good thing, too.
- **On-all-fours 69.** In a more traditional 69, one partner lays down while the other partner gets on top on all fours while they both give and receive. This position can potentially provide a bit more "breathing room" than facesitting and can be a nice set-up for mutual pleasure.

- **Make it extra tasty**. Although vulvas are already often tasty on their own, some people enjoy adding flavor to their vulva for the sake of variety or pleasure. Though this is not recommended for women who are prone to yeast infections or other forms of vaginal or vulvar irritation, other women may enjoy spraying whipped cream, sprinkling body sugar, or slathering flavored lube on their genital parts. The safest place for these tasty playthings is farther away from the vaginal entrance, such as on the mons, the outer labia, and the top of the clitoris, such as around the clitoral hood. However, if you're irritation-prone, you may want to skip this altogether. As always, if you have questions about your personal health or what is or is not safe for you, check in with your healthcare provider.

INTERCOURSE? OF COURSE!

Although there are numerous sex positions that can be found in books—or your imagination—sometimes the most pleasurable positions involve slight modifications of old stand-bys. Here are a few ways to transform common sex positions into uncommon pleasure.

Mission: Pleasure Possible

When some people hear "missionary," they think of boring, awkward, fumbling sex. But missionary is perhaps the most common sex position for a reason—namely, it can be an easy sex position in which a woman can relax and focus on her pleasure and orgasm. Try these adaptations that may stimulate your vulva or vagina in more targeted ways:

- **Tilt your hips upward during missionary, making your torso as flat as a table.** If your partner's penis or strap-on points or aims upward, this can aid in G-spot stimulation. Downward pointing or side-to-side play can also be fun. Squeeze your pelvic-floor muscles (the muscles that help draw your vagina in tighter) for more intense stimulation for yourself and your partner. You might also find it easier to place a pillow under your hips so that you can relax rather than holding your hips up with your own strength.

- **Become a CAT lady.** CAT stands for coital alignment technique, another modification of missionary. Have your male partner (or your female partner if she's wearing a strap-on) position their shoulders past yours, closer to your ears or forehead. This should allow your partner's pubic bone to more easily rub against your vulva. This placement combined with the motions—which are more about close grinding than in and out thrusting—has been shown to make for easier orgasms for women.[11–14]

Breaking the Sex Ceiling: Woman on Top

Although woman on top is another popular sex position (at least in part due to Sharon Stone's sexy ways in the movie *Basic Instinct*), many women aren't sure what to do once they get on top. In fact, this is a question that Debby has been asked hundreds of times in her work as a sex educator and columnist. Here are four possibilities—though you should feel free to get creative all on your own.

- **Top a squat.** Plant one foot flat on the ground on either side of your partner's torso, with your knees facing forward or out to the sides (if you have knee problems or concerns about your knee health or safety, check in with your healthcare provider before trying this or any other sex position that works or puts stress on your knees). Using your hands on your partner's torso or on the bed for leverage, rise up to slide your vagina up the shaft of your partner's penis or strap-on and then back down. Squeeze your pelvic-floor muscles for more intense stimulation.

- **Lean forward.** Whether your feet or knees are planted on either side of your partner, leaning forward allows you to get closer to your partner, which can allow for kissing and building intimacy. If your partner's penis or strap-on points or bends upward, this can also intensify G-Spot stimulation for you.
- **Lean back.** No matter which way your partner points or bends, leaning back can stimulate the front vaginal wall (G-spot area), as everything your partner's got down there will be pressing against that front vaginal wall. Leaning back also makes it easier for your partner to stimulate your clitoris with his/her fingers or a sex toy, such as a vibrator.
- **Grind it.** Slowly move your hips forward and back, grinding your partner's genitals. Then try moving your hips in circles, thus providing ample stimulation to your entire vulva.

Of course, you can also turn around and try these reverse cowgirl style, facing your partner's feet.

Back It On Up: Rear Entry

Sometimes people think of rear entry between a man and a woman as being more about the man's pleasure than the woman's pleasure. After all, rear entry can be a pretty deep-thrusting position, which can mean that a woman's cervix gets bumped up against (pleasurable for some women, but uncomfortable or painful for others). Rear-entry sex positions (a.k.a. doggie style) have also gotten a bad rap thanks to their frequent presence in, well, rap. Although sex as portrayed in some rap and hip-hop songs has shaped many women's sexuality in positive ways, there are also a number of lyrics and videos that have made some women feel more objectified than respected as an equal partner in pleasure—and all too often, doggie style has been used as a part of those messages. Nevertheless, rear entry can be a pleasurable part of many women's sex lives. Here are two ways to make it work in your favor:

QUIRKY QUEEFS

If you've ever had a moment of passing air through your vagina in a kind of noisy way—perhaps during sex—you may have wondered what the heck happened. Vaginal queefs (also called varts, vaginal farts, vaginal flatulence, and fanny farts) aren't farts at all—meaning, they don't involve passing gas and thus aren't smelly. Rather, a queef involves trapped air passing out of the vagina. Some women experience queefs during exercise, such as sit-ups. More often, they're heard during sex. Queefs are very common—especially in conjunction with vigorous thrusting sex positions that move air in and out of the vagina—and nothing to be embarrassed about. What are the rules of eti-queefe-tte? There really are none. We recommend that you just laugh and move on.

- **All fours.** This is traditional doggie style in which a woman is on all fours while her partner thrusts while kneeling or standing behind her. You can keep your back flat as a table for moderate-depth thrusting or lean down, with your head in the pillows, for deeper thrusting (this poses a greater likelihood of bumping against the cervix, so proceed with caution). If your partner is particularly large or you find the depth of thrusting uncomfortable, ask him to wear a two-holed masturbation sleeve on his penis. Sleeves with a hole at each end can be slipped over his penis and squished down to the base, giving him total coverage (the toy stimulates the bottom half and you stimulate the top half) while you don't have to take as much in at a time.
- **Lay down.** Once you two are "inserted" in the all-fours position, you may find it pleasurable to keep your bodies connected as you slink downward and lay on the bed on your

stomach. If your partner pops out, try raising your hips upward for easier re-entry. By laying down for rear entry, you can minimize the thrusting pace and depth, which can be easier on your vagina and cervix. Women who enjoy G-spot or clitoral stimulation may also find this pleasurable, as they can grind against their partner and their bed, while face-down.

ANOTHER V WORTH CELEBRATING: VIBRATORS!

Many women are curious about vibrators. In fact, according to research that our team published in 2009, 53 percent of women and nearly half of men have used a vibrator. Most men who had used a vibrator had done so with a partner, though nearly one out of five had tried vibrator play alone.[15] Here's your opportunity for a crash course on vibrators for vivacious vaginal and vulvar play (how's that for a bunch of Vs?), including how to choose vibrators and other sex toys and how to put them to good, and possibly orgasmic, use.

In her work as a sex educator and columnist, Debby is often asked how to choose a vibrator that's good for beginners. While there is no one vibrator that will be right for everyone, here are a few things to keep in mind. A woman who is new to vibrators and other sex toys might be best served to choose one that:

- **Delivers the kind of stimulation she knows that she enjoys.** For example, women who prefer G-spot stimulation might want to choose a vibrator that can be inserted into the vagina for G-spot play.
- **Has variable speeds.** After all, if you've never used a vibrator before, the only way to know if you like light stimulation or very intense stimulation is to choose one that has multiple speeds, preferably one with a multi-speed dial rather than a toy with pre-set buttons that delivers certain intensities. That

way, you can have more control over the degree of stimulation you want to try.

- **Is easy to clean.** This means that the toy should have few crevices and preferably come with cleaning instructions or information from a knowledgeable sales clerk at a sex boutique, in-home sex-toy party, or through information at a reputable web site (see Resources).
- **Is affordable.** Vibrator play should be pleasurable. If you've spent more than you can afford, you may be less likely to relax, let go, and enjoy the experience. Until you know what kind of vibrator you really like, stick with a less costly model that is well within your budget.
- **Is safe.** Try to choose a toy made of non-toxic, non-porous materials, such as glass or medical-grade silicone. Though silicone toys can be more expensive than Jelly toys, they tend to be safer and easier to clean and are often available at affordable price points (as are many glass vibrators and non-vibrating dildos).

If you have one of the following sex toys (some of which are vibrators, though not all are), consider these tips on pleasurable vulva and vagina play.

- **Vaginal vibrators** may be long, smooth, and almost cylindrical, or they may be shaped like a penis (some even have features that look like veins in the shaft and a scrotum). Vaginal vibrators are particularly good choices for women who enjoy vaginal stimulation and/or G-spot stimulation. You may want to choose a vaginal vibrator with a tapered end, as all too often the head of the vibrator is too large for comfortable insertion—even with exciting build-up and lubricant.
- **Non-vibrating dildos** are basically like vaginal vibrators but without the vibration. They too may resemble a penis (or not).

More and more often, dildos are being made with non-toxic materials, such as glass or hardwood. Again, you'll want to choose a shaft that can comfortably fit inside your vagina. One variation on dildos is the double dildo, which is well suited for sex play between two women. If you're shopping for a dildo to use in a harness, you'll want to make sure that it can fit inside the harness in a stable manner so that it doesn't move around too much during sex play. Some harnesses come with dildos; if yours doesn't, you may find it helpful to ask a knowledgeable store clerk if she recommends a certain dildo to go with your harness type.

- **G-spot toys** may be vibrating or non-vibrating. The chief difference is that they are curved for easier stimulation of the front vaginal wall.
- **Clitoral vibrators** are some of the most commonly used types of sex toys. Although many women enjoy vaginal pen-etration, our research suggests that more women use vibrators to stimulate their clitoris than the vagina. Popular clitoral models include the silver bullet and egg varieties, which can be found at most adult bookstores, sex boutiques, sex-toy web sites, and in-home sex-toy party companies. Clitoral-focused vibrators have an advantage in that they tend to be small and thus easier to use during vaginal intercourse with a partner, as they can slip easily in between partners' bodies.
- **Double-duty vibrators** are sometimes called "dual action vibrators." These models usually provide possibilities to stim-ulate the clitoris and vagina at the same time. The Rabbit is one of the more famous double-duty vibrators thanks to an appearance on *Sex and the City*. Look for a model that allows you to operate each part independently. That way, you can turn the clitoral vibrator on while leaving the vaginal vibrator off or vice versa.
- **Triple-duty vibrators** are sometimes more difficult to find in stores. They offer clitoral, vaginal, and anal stimulation.

- **Vaginal balls (also called Ben Wa balls)** don't vibrate, but they're an interesting sexual-enhancement aid in that they can be used for pleasure or for vaginal health (see chapter 2 for more information on Kegel exercises). Some women insert vaginal balls into their vagina and squeeze their pelvic-floor muscles to stimulate themselves as part of masturbation. Ben Wa balls and Smart Balls are among the types of vaginal balls that are widely available.

- **Vibrating c-rings** can be worn around a man's penis. The ring puts slight constrictive pressure on a man's penis and may feel pleasurable. Along one part of the ring, there is sometimes a small, bullet-like vibrator that, if worn on top of the shaft during face-to-face sex (such as missionary), may be well positioned to stimulate a woman's clitoris. Note: a c-ring (also called a cock ring or penis ring) is generally not recommended for use for longer than twenty minutes at a time. It should also be removed if a man finds it uncomfortable or if he's had experiences with penile bruising or pain from wearing such rings.

TEST YOUR VQ

1. The clitoral complex is composed of all of the following EXCEPT the
   a. vagina
   b. urethra
   c. labia
   d. clitoris

2. A woman may experience orgasm as a result of sensory information from which of the following nerves:
   a. pudendal nerve
   b. pelvic nerve
   c. hypogastric nerve
   d. vagus nerve
   e. all of the above

3. According to data from the National Survey of Sexual Health and Behavior (NSSHB), approximately how many women experienced difficulty with lubrication during their most recent experience having sex?
   a. 5 percent
   b. 10 percent
   c. 30 percent
   d. 50 percent

Answers

1. c
2. e
3. c

• 4 •

How Do I Look?

How We Come to Think and Feel the Way We Do about Our Vulvas

I'LL SHOW YOU MINE IF YOU SHOW ME YOURS

$\mathcal{A}$s a young child, did you ever play "doctor"? Or games like "I'll show you mine if you show me yours"? If so, you're not alone. A number of research studies—including a study that Debby worked on years ago when she first began working at The Kinsey Institute—have found that young children (both girls and boys) play games like this.[1] It's a common way that girls and boys learn about their bodies and explore the world around them.

A particularly interesting study on this topic was conducted in Germany by Dr. Bettine Schuhrke.[2] She studied children at age two and again at age six to understand how they came to learn about their genitals. Specifically, she asked one parent of each child in the study (typically she asked the mother) to answer questions about the various ways that their child had indicated an interest in their own or another's genitals. She found that, at the age of two, over 90 percent of the children had behaved in a way that indicated an interest in another person's genitals (e.g., the genitals of the child's mother, father, brother, sister, etc.). In her research article, Dr. Schuhrke provided an example of a toddler who noticed her father's penis as he was changing one day. The toddler asked to touch it and her father allowed her to. The toddler continued to ask every day for about a week and a half before she lost interest in her father's penis. Although this is an example of a girl learning about male genitals, the young girls in the study were equally as interested in learning about the vulva.

Another interesting finding is that children in this study typically only began to explore and ask questions about other people's genitals after they had already explored their own. Why is this important? First of all, if you have or care for children now or in the future, we want you to feel prepared for some very common situations of general exploration. There's no reason to feel alarmed if, for instance, your child points to your genitals or asks questions about your genitals while you're going to the bathroom, taking a shower, or changing clothes. Second, and more importantly, we want to reassure you that this is totally and completely 100 percent normal. Genital curiosity begins at a stage before most children are even able to contemplate the complications of playing doctor or house. And if children are exposed to family members of another sex, then they often want to know why their private parts look different from their own. All of this is a normal part of how young humans learn about bodies.

Cunt-parisons

Given how common it is for children to explore their own genitals and those of other children, you might wonder what happens to this genital curiosity as children get older. Some children don't do much exploring for years. They may be satisfied with having learned about the differences between boys' bodies and girls' bodies, or they may have been scolded for touching their own genitals or those of a friend and feel scared or embarrassed to touch themselves or ask to see another child's body again. Other children continue their exploration. As children become more "sex-segregated"—meaning that girls tend to play mostly with other girls and boys tend to play mostly with other boys—some of this genital curiosity turns into genital comparison. Women in our research studies have talked about comparing their vulvas, and specifically their labia, with their friends. Also, in her book *Chelsea Chelsea Bang Bang*, comedian and author Chelsea Handler wrote about learning to masturbate at a sleepover at a childhood friend's home.[3] Like teenagers and adults, children compare bodies and genitals both because they are curious and also because they want to know if they are "normal."

As a professional dancer early on in my career (I was perhaps 20), I was in a show where everyone was super comfortable and we were always naked in our dressing room. I remember some of my friends comparing labia one day and for me, I had never stared so closely or had such an up close look at a vagina other than mine. I found it fascinating. I loved seeing how different they all were. I haven't had much opportunity since then (aside from porn) as my partners have all been men.

—KATE, 28, Canada

For many other body parts, the "am I normal?" question is an easy one to answer. If we want to know whether our ears are large or small, all we have to do is look around at other people's ears. After all, ears are everywhere and easily seen. The same is true for noses, butts, and even—to some extent—breasts (though it's not always so easy to tell what's real or not due to padded/enhanced bras and breast implants). From these comparisons, we can usually identify where we fit along the spectrum of height, weight, breast size, nose size, ear size, and so on. We may not be thrilled with what we notice, but at least people have a sense of where they belong and the knowledge that others are like them.

Vulvas are an entirely different story. How are girls or women supposed to know what other vulvas look like? Vulvas are not noses or even breasts. Even in leggings or bathing suits it can be tricky to see any genital detail. When we've asked this question to groups of men, they often are quick to suggest that there are plenty of opportunities for women to compare and contrast genitals, frequently citing the locker room as a good place to get a sense of what other women's genitals look like. Those of us who spend time at the gym know that's not the case, though. First, it feels creepy and inappropriate to stare at other women's genitals when uninvited. Second, few women parade around the gym completely nude. In our gym experiences, women seem to spend only a short amount of time naked before putting their clothes back on. And third, even when women are nude, there's rarely much that one can see. Pubic hair, for those who keep it, conceals some parts of the vulva. Also, unless a woman parts her legs, there's not often a lot to see. Vulva parts are naturally kind of "hidden" between a woman's legs.

The first real one I saw was my sister's—when she needed me to help her apply some medication. I was surprised, and I think pleased, that hers and mine looked so similar.

—MAGGIE, 61, California

If women aren't able to get a sense of what other women's vulvas look like from being in locker rooms or other public spaces, then what opportunities do women have to learn what's common or not when it comes to vulvas? Friends? Perhaps. Some women may compare genitals with friends. Lovers? Yes, but this is only true if a woman has a sexual partner who also has a vulva. Even for the minority of women who do have female sexual partners, they may only have a limited number of female partners, thus giving them a limited view of the diverse range of vulvas in the world.

So, how are women supposed to know which genitals look "normal"? For all women, the story is likely a little different. We have both found that the vulva pictures that we show in classes or presentations are sometimes the first images of vulvas that women have ever seen (including their own). Other women have seen the vulvas of friends, lovers, or family members. Yet, those women who are curious about the appearance of women's genitals who don't have access to other women's genitals may seek out the information from a variety of other sources.

WHEREFORE ART THOU, LABIA?

If you were curious about the appearance of women's genitals, where would be the best place to look? We are not sure where you should look, but we certainly know where you should *not* look. Psychologist Ros Bramwell[4] at the University of Liverpool investigated a variety of "glossy" women's magazines in search of pictures with a visible pubic area. These magazines were not the kind that you would have to request from behind a counter or extract from a protective clear plastic cover with "warning signs" for explicit material. These magazines were the kind that you might leaf through while standing in line at the checkout counter at your local grocery store—in other words, mainstream women's lifestyle and fashion magazines.

In these magazines, Bramwell[4] and a research assistant extracted all pictures of women with a visible pubic area including pictures of models in bathing suits, underwear, tight-fitting clothing, and, of course, nude. From 240 pictures that fit these criteria, they analyzed the 49 pictures that did not require a magnifying glass to view the up-close details. From those pictures, they eliminated all pictures that obscured the model's pubic area with shading, bulky clothing, crossed legs, and so on. In this final set of pictures, they looked closely at the model's pubic area for bumps, humps, or other lady lumps. They reviewed many magazines and used a rigorous scientific method. Even without opening a magazine, we bet that you can guess what they found. If you guessed "nothing," you would be correct. They didn't notice any protruding labia. They found a surprising number of pictures (six pictures, or 14 percent of all pictures with a visible pubic area) that showed an "extrusion or indentation." However, their description of these pictures was "of tight clothing being drawn up between the labia majora,"[4] which sounds like a formal description of camel-toe to us. We were not surprised by the lack of definable genitalia in these magazines. Sure, European magazines tend to be a bit more relaxed about nudity, but they were still mainstream magazines

PAPER MACHE PANTY PARTY

Panty party: sounds like something that would spontaneously break out during an all-girl sleepover following a really rambunctious pillow fight. Not quite, but it is designed to be a female bonding experience. Plus, the original French phrase, *papier mâché* (say "mah-shay"), means "chewed paper," which we like because, if you think of the vagina dentata myth (the idea that vaginas have teeth), it's kind of an interesting coincidence, yes? In English, it's written as "paper mache."

What You Need

- One pair of panties per person. They can be fierce, hideous, or lovely. They can be thongs or high-waisted bloomers. There are no rules on the types of panties you can use. Genitals come in all shapes and sizes and so should the range of panties!
- Newspapers, magazines, or printed pictures/words (try to use old paper to recycle). Newspapers work best, but magazines can work with enough patience.
- water
- flour or glue (the regular white sticky stuff)
- mixing bowl
- mixer (optional)
- balloons
- hairdryer (optional)
- paint
- decorations (Be Creative! We love sequins, feathers, and rhinestones.)
- clothesline and pins (optional)

Directions

1. Get your group together. This is a great activity for a group of ladies, but there is no harm in involving the fellas. Consider a panty party in lieu of your next couple's game night. The point of the party is to get a conversation and celebration started. So

decide on a group that will help make that happen. You can provide the panties and decorations if you are concerned about over-burdening your guests. However, the party is designed to celebrate diversity, and there is no better way to do that than by asking your guests to bring the items that represent their individuality!

2. Begin the party by asking everyone to tear off adjectives, words, or images that express how they feel or would like to feel about their genitals. The strips should be about one inch by one inch. As you all tear, discuss what words/images you are choosing and why. If you want a themed paper-mache panty, consider printing a variety of different words or vulva images. If you want to save your guests time, you can also consider doing this beforehand.

3. Time for everyone to get their panties in a bunch! That's right; everyone sets up panty workstations. This is where the balloons come in (and you thought they were just for celebration). Blow up the balloon a little bit to give it some initial shape. Now stick it inside the panty and continue to blow it up until it gives the panty a full shape. The balloons are going to hold the panties in place while you paper mache.

4. Mix one part water to two parts glue, if you decided to use glue, or one part flour with two parts water, if you are using flour. If you are using flour, mix it together until it is smooth and not bumpy. It can get messy, so you may want to make a few different mixtures to reduce the amount of dripping.

5. Let the fun begin! Dip the pieces of paper into the mixture, making sure all sides are completely covered. Pull off excess mixture by running the paper through your fingers. Stick the paper pieces onto the panties, curling them underneath the edges to follow the shape of the panty. Continue until the panties have one layer of paper.

6. Wait for the first layer to dry. You can expedite this process by using a hairdryer. Complete at least two more layers to make sure that it maintains its shape. Always make sure the layer is completely dry before adding another one.

> 7. Once the final product is dry, it is time to decorate! Have some negative words or pictures on the panties? It is your time to cover them up with paint. Choose colors that represent how you feel about your genitals. Snazz them up by decorating with buttons, sequins, or feathers. Get creative!
> 8. Have an organization or institution that you think would benefit from a vulva-awareness art project? If so, hang the finished projects on a clothesline to remind everyone that their vulva is beautiful and unique.

where airbrushing and other digital editing of photos are the norm and genital (or any) bumps/lumps are quickly wiped away.

I wish there was more education on the variations of colour, sizes, symmetry etc. so women don't feel like they're abnormal. Where I come from it's illegal to show unedited pictures of vulvas in magazines. It's stupid and the reason why most of the vulvas I saw were cartoons/drawings.

—KARA, 20, Tonga

It was disappointing to us that there were no depictions of defined genitalia in mainstream "glossy" magazines, but it was not entirely surprising; it can be tricky to see genital definition through women's clothing. We had to wonder, what about pictures of women without clothing? How are those women's genitals portrayed?

The Playboy Perspective

While in graduate school, Vanessa and two colleagues (Sarah Calabrese and Brandi Rima) decided that a content analysis of sexually explicit materials was in order.[5] The question was, where to begin? Although sexually explicit materials have probably been around since the beginning of mankind, stone carvings always left much to the imagination. Even paintings were simply a rendition of the artist's view of the woman. Then, there was Hugh. Hugh Hefner mainstreamed nude images of women in 1953 with the introduction of *Playboy*, which boasted a wonderfully voluptuous, debatably size-12 Marilyn Monroe on the first cover.[6-9]

Since that original cover with Marilyn Monroe, a lot has changed. Poodle skirts went out of style, bras were burned, and leg warmers became all the rage. Just as there have been women's clothing trends that have come and gone, there have also been changes in women's bodies (or at least the ways in which women's bodies have been portrayed) underneath all that clothing. Consequently, Vanessa and her colleagues set out to conduct an empirical investigation of these trends using rigorous and scientific methods. They gathered every centerfold picture (from 1953 to the most recent issue at the time in 2007) and set about looking for trends in women's body size and shape over time. Because they all came into the project with theories about how the models would change over time, an objective way to understand the ways that models' bodies changed over time (or did not) needed to be developed. In order to do this, they decided that they couldn't be the ones who evaluated the centerfold models and found a few open-minded students who were interested in helping with the project. Next, the research assistants were trained on what to look for.

The first part was easy, as the models' body measurements (breast, waist, and hip size, along with height and weight) are listed next to each one of the pictures. If you are reading this and yelling, "Girl, if I was asked to list my measurements in that magazine there is NO WAY that I would report my accurate measurements!" then you are in good company. (Vanessa has tried to give herself a few inches of height on her driver's license every renewal year without any success.) Needless to say, we thought the same thing. So, how do we know the measurements listed are accurate, then? We don't, and in fact, we would be surprised if they were. The research team made peace with this because the important thing wasn't whether the model from January 1982 had larger breasts or a thinner waist than the model of May 1968. Women's average breast size probably changes very little from decade to decade, so if the model said her breasts were a little bigger one year and a little smaller during the next few years, that was more interesting because it demonstrated a trend in cultural ideals of beauty. In other words, if women were fudging their measurements, we were interested in whether they were making the measurements bigger or smaller each year.

Next, the team had to decide on how to evaluate changes in women's genitals. Unlike body-size measurements, there were no details listed about the models' pubic hair length or labia size. The team had to ask themselves how much pubic hair could be missing before they considered the model to be "shaved" (waxed, electrolysized, etc.)? What would be considered "longer" inner labia, and what should be considered "shorter" inner labia? These were not easy questions to answer and required Vanessa and her research team to spend many long and tedious (but joyful) evenings debating these philosophical questions. They would come up with a set of criteria, and then two of them would evaluate a set of pictures. The next day they would come together and talk through how everyone had scored each picture. They did this again . . . and again . . . and again until finally, they were in almost 100 percent agreement. A few gray hairs later, they were finally ready to give the categories to the research assistants who would separately code the models' pubic hair and genital appearance in an objective manner. As one final safeguard, the centerfold images were shuffled so that the research assistants wouldn't know which models belonged to which years.

What did Vanessa and her team find? In the 1950s and early 1960s, they saw models with curvaceous frames, demure poses, big updos, large round breasts, and concealed genitals (most would turn their back or cross their legs, making the genitals difficult or impossible to see). The late 1960s and 1970s brought a sexual revolution along with a more natural-looking model characterized by straight hair and a curly bush down below, sometimes referred to as a "fur bikini" because of the ability of natural pubic hair to hide genital details such as the labia. The models of the 1980s got a little taller (about half an inch) and thinner (about 2.5 pounds) than those in earlier years. However, little changed south of the border. Over 95 percent of the models in the magazine in the 1970s and 1980s displayed seemingly natural pubic hair (e.g., pubic hair that had not been removed). That said, likely due to advancements in plastic surgery in the 1980s and 1990s, the average model's breasts were about an inch larger than a decade earlier. As the models' breasts grew, their pubic hair began to disappear. Over a third of the models in the 1990s appear to have modified their pubic hair (although few removed it completely). If that seems like a lot, then get this: that number more than doubled during the twenty-first century, when less than 10 percent of the women wore their pubic hair au natural. The most popular style was to remove the hair partially (over two-thirds of the women), but a new "style" also began making an appearance: approximately a quarter of the women were bare down there.

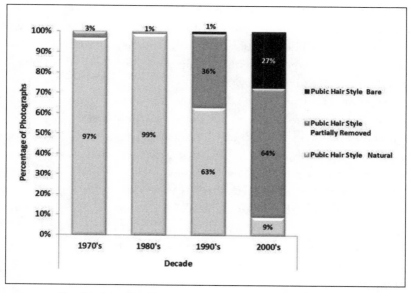

Trends in Pubic Hair Patterns by Decade in a Popular Men's Magazine

Going Bare

Do you ever wonder what your head would look like if you shaved off all your hair? Some women do, especially when they are facing treatments (such as chemotherapy) that result in hair loss. But most of the time, women probably don't spend too much time thinking about what their scalp would look like without hair. After all, unless you've experienced hair loss for medical reasons or are among the minority of women who choose to shave it all off, the scalp is rarely seen, except perhaps by one's hair stylist or an attentive lover who brushes one's hair or massages one's head.

However, what if Sinead O'Connor had another hit and head-shaving became all the rage? Would you then wonder whether you had an "attractive" head? Would you wonder what characteristics distinguish between an attractive and unattractive head? We wonder if these kinds of discussions came up regarding vulvas when pubic hair started disappearing and vulvas became more visible than ever before. And if these discussions did come up, did someone decide that they weren't going to show long inner labia anymore, now that there was no pubic hair to hide the vulva parts? Or is there another reason why inner labia are largely absent, or minimized, in some mainstream men's magazines such as *Playboy*?

Unfortunately, we don't know the answers to these questions. What we do know is that inner labia were only visible in a small handful of the images that Vanessa's research team examined. Also, not a single image showed inner labia that protruded beyond the outer labia or that were a color other than pink.

These results were surprising to Vanessa and her team. They went in expecting that there wouldn't be a lot of inner labia shown protruding—but none? How could that be? After all, the world is full of women with long, beautiful labia (and the men and women in another one of our research studies sometimes cited a preference for long labia).

I'm tired of the societal/media/porn industry pressure on women to have "perfect" genitals. It needs to stop! I think that it's sick that women are going under the knife to alter themselves. We need to stop the hate!

—MARY, 35, Washington, DC

Not wanting to jump to any conclusions, the research team wondered whether this was perhaps just a reflection of the centerfold models. Would the other models in the magazine look any different? In a follow-up study, they examined each picture from the most recent year of *Playboy*. They categorized every picture of a woman who wasn't wearing underwear. Again, they found that over 90 percent of the pictures did not show any inner labia. Also, there were only two images of protruding labia and one lone image of inner labia that was a color other than pink (and even that picture was possibly just showing a shadow). Sure, some women don't have very visible inner labia, many women's labia do not protrude, and lots of women have pink inner labia, but the likelihood that every single one of these women happened to have identical vulvas is very slim. There was certainly something wrong with these pictures!

Vulva Education

Whenever Vanessa discusses these results at a scientific conference, she makes the point that one reason this is important is because many young women and men see their very first vulvas when they look at magazines like *Playboy*. While a quick glimpse at the world around them will let them know that women aren't normally as skinny as *Playboy* models and don't often have the same figures, one can't just glimpse around to see that even the vulvas don't add up. As such, *Playboy* and other mainstream men's magazines may misinform women and men about what's "normal" for women in terms of their genitals. Because people want to feel normal, this is important.

When she makes this point, Vanessa often gets the same question:

What about other sources for genital images? After all, women may seek out genital images from a variety of different sources. Some may look in magazines, and others may seek out anatomy textbooks in their local libraries. Given how private people feel about genitals (some even call them their "privates"), it is less likely that people are openly seeking out these images when they have access to a plethora of vulva images on their home computer.

Time and again people have tried to tell us that women should not be concerned about their vulva appearance because they have a variety of vulva images available to them at the click of a button. The only problem is the type of images that pop up for the uninformed vulva investigator. Let us demonstrate. Put on your savvy vulva sleuth hat for a second and pull up your preferred Internet search engine. After you have checked to make sure that your computer is up-to-date on pop-up blockers and firewalls, type the word "vagina" or "vulva" into your search engine. What pops up? A beautiful, diverse range of vulva pictures? Unlikely. Chances are that you—like us—came across a lot of internal diagrams, several web sites about cancer, a few pornographic web sites, and an advertisement for elective genital surgery. Now try it again, this time searching only for images. Again, you are unlikely to have any luck. When we tried this, the images and messages were the same, with the exception of a few pictures of animal vulvas, which—not surprisingly—can be quite misleading!

Vulva Close-ups

Even if you decide to weed through Internet pornography for a diverse range of vulva images, you may not find what you're looking for. A recent study[10] sought to investigate whether the range of vulva appearances presented in textbooks, books designed to represent vulva diversity (which they termed "feminist publications"), and pornographic web sites were significantly different from one another. They took measurements of the vulvas of the women represented in these three sources by literally measuring the clitoral hood length, inner and outer labia length, and distance from the clitoral hood to the urethra. In order to get the measurement for the protrusion of the inner labia from the outer labia, the researchers guesstimated using a five-point scale with every point indicating a ten-millimeter protuberance.

BETTY DODSON'S GENITAL IMAGE GALLERY

Betty Dodson has worked tirelessly for more than thirty-five years to bring vulva pride to women everywhere. She has done many wonderful things that will forever change the way many women think about their bodies. Our personal favorite is her online genital art gallery. If you go to her web site (now shared with the delightful Carlin Ross) at www.dodsonandross.com, you can easily find her genital art galleries. Betty started this online gallery a while back to provide men and women with a platform to submit their own genital pictures and write about the reasons why they love them. These images likely served many purposes for many people; however, the primary intention was to provide real images of the vast range of normal/natural genital appearances. Due to some legal changes, people can still submit photographs to the site, but they can no longer be anonymous. The web site is now required to ask for identification confirming a user's age before he or she can post genital pictures. If you are less interested in submitting a picture and more interested in browsing the pictures, this is a top pick. For other wonderful web sites with diverse vulva images, check out the Resources section.

When first reading this study, we were wary about the results because we were not entirely clear how they controlled for the fact that the pictures may have been taken at different distances or from different angles. After further reflection, we realized that the measurements are not meant to reflect *actual* vulva measurements of the women; they are meant to represent depictions of the vulva to readers who may be viewing the images.

Keeping that disclaimer in mind, the researchers found that the pictures showed the least diversity in the textbook images (and this is where we are supposed to learn!), followed by online pornography, with the most variation evident in "feminist resources." Pictures of labia that protruded to their highest measurement of protrusion were only available in the feminist resources. What does that mean? On the bright side, it means that there are several resources for women who are interested in viewing a range of genital images. In the study, they analyzed two of our personal favorite collections of vulva images: *Petals* by Nick Karras[11] and *Femalia* by Joani Blank.[12] On the other hand, it

---

SEXUAL ASSAULT: STORIES OF RESILIENCE

This book was intended to be a celebration of all of the wonders of the vulva. The vulva has many amazing characteristics including its ability to clean itself, open and lubricate for pleasurable experiences, and perhaps most importantly, bring human life into this world. As undeniably phenomenal as each one of these features is, it is the experiences and the resilience of the women who own these vulvas and vaginas that we found truly awe-inspiring.

Every woman's relationship and experience with her genitals is different. Some women have always loved their bodies, while others are still searching for self-love. There are also those women who are hoping to reclaim, or who have reclaimed, the genital love that they may have felt was lost following sexual trauma. The experience of each and every woman is unique, but we hope that the following stories will inspire you to continue your search or support someone else along her journey toward genital love and acceptance.

"I was raped by my father when I was four years old. That changed my attitude about my yoni from natural acceptance to hatred. I came to like myself again when I discovered female ejaculation, sex-positive people, and BDSM. I learned to explore without judgment and won my curiosity back."—Patricia, Washington

"I felt ashamed of my genitals as a child. I came to feel positively about my genitals by visiting feminist/sex-positive/body-positive health web sites as an adolescent when I was looking for informa-

also means that women who are seeking out information regarding the normal range of vulva appearances may have a skewed representation of "normal" if they are getting their information from another source.

THE (W)HOLE TRUTH

Some resources show vulvas with small labia, some show large labia, and some don't show any at all (there is a Goldilocks reference in

tion. Reading through the web sites reassured me that my vulva and vagina were 'normal.' Learning about my anatomy and getting my questions answered made me feel less shame. These web sites also helped after being assaulted, because I realized that the physical consequences I experienced were normal and not my fault. That was a huge relief. After my assault, I've also come to feel more 'ownership' over my genitals—that is, as the feelings of shame went away, I felt more and more 'in charge' of my own body, and I think I value or cherish it more now. I've made a conscious effort to avoid criticizing my vagina or vulva's appearance or function."—Sarah, 22, Wisconsin

"I'm a strong feminist. Before realizing this, I just pretended my vagina/vulva didn't exist. And then felt immensely guilty for wanting to use it sexually. Because women aren't supposed to be the gender with strong sexual desire. Purportedly. However, I just finished my third year of the vagina monologues, and have recovered from rape. Part of that self-discovery and healing process come with loving yourself. And a major symbolic and very real part of myself is my vagina. I'm still working on it, and I backslide, but the consciousness is there."—Melissa, 21, Washington

"Although I was raped in high school it never affected my feelings about my vagina, only my self-esteem. I know this is different for many women and I feel extremely lucky. I am now, however, very sensitive to when and when not I am ok with being touched, and more able to express that."—Karen, 20, Washington

there somewhere). Why does it matter? The same can be said for most body portrayals in mainstream magazines that tend to feature size 0 models in their teens or early twenties. The difference with vulvas is that we all know that pictures of the models in magazines do not look like the women that we see on the streets every day. There are a select few women who fit that profile, and even those women have been airbrushed to be suitable for presentation in the magazines. We know this because (a) we can see it, and (b) we can talk about it. In contrast, unless you are living in a nudist colony or visiting a clothing-optional beach, you are probably not surrounded by images of women's genitals. Those women with questions or concerns about the appearance of their vulvas may consider the matter too private or embarrassing to discuss with others. As such, when women see these vulva images in magazines or textbooks, they may automatically use them as a reference point for what vulvas should look like. If the appearance of their own vulvas deviates from those images, these women may become concerned that the appearance of their vulvas is not normal or that it is unattractive.

This can be both good news and bad news. The bad news is that a lot of women may rely on these restricted genital resources for information; the good news is that there are other resources that show a diverse range of vulva images. We were curious whether these images actually impacted the way women viewed their vulvas.

OUR LABIA, OURSELVES

Vanessa and a team of researchers at George Washington University conducted two experiments (and we are both in the process of conducting a third at Indiana University) to investigate this question.[13] As researchers, we are always excited when we come across a new unanswered question to investigate. We keep several tools in our toolboxes for such occasions including surveys, experiments, observations, and interviews. Although any of these methods would have helped us answer our question of interest, conducting an actual experiment can help the researcher maintain control over the kinds of information available to the participants, and this can yield more easily interpretable results. Consequently, Vanessa set about designing an experiment. In the first experiment, female college students were randomly assigned to one of four different groups. Participants in the first three groups were asked to rate a series of six vulva pictures. The first group saw pictures of airbrushed vulvas from a popular men's magazine, the second group saw pictures of vulvas after labiaplasty (an elective procedure for labia reductions), and the third group saw the vulvas of the exact same women before they underwent labiaplasty (their "before" photos). The fourth group did not see any pictures at all. The participants were also asked several questions about the appearance of their vulva including how large/small various components were, what their ideal vulva would look like, and how satisfied they were with various components of their vulva. Approximately two hundred female undergraduate students participated in the online experiment. Participants had no idea that they had been assigned to a certain group and would be seeing different images than the next participant in line.

The day that data came back, the first thing Vanessa was interested in was whether the women rated one picture set as significantly more attractive than the others. They had, without a doubt, rated the men's magazine pictures the most attractive.[13] While this may feel disappointing for all of us who do not have runway model vulvas, we have to keep in mind that those pictures were the only ones that were airbrushed. It is quite possible that the participants were responding to the nice airbrushed quality that we have become accustomed to by reading magazines. In addition to rating the mainstream men's magazines as the most attractive, most participants also indicated that their ideal vulva would be "smaller." Of course, not all stated this, but that was the trend. Finally, the key question was, given that we knew that these women thought smaller, airbrushed vulvas were more ideal, how did viewing these pictures make them feel about their own vulvas?

Before guessing, think about the last time you opened a fashion magazine and looked at the models. How did you feel about your body? Now, take a look around the locker room, subway station, or wherever you come across "ordinary" women. Have your feelings about your body changed? It is likely that they have, just as they did for the women in the study.

I only learned—in the last five years—that women have different vaginas— protruding inner labia, etc. I don't think that women see enough images of vulvas. They are airbrushed in skin mags and considered pornographic. I think that hinders women's pride in their genitals.

—JOY, 40, Australia

After taking into consideration factors like the frequency with which the women in the study looked at pornography, how frequently they engaged in sexual behavior with other women, how often they checked out their own lady bits, and so on, Vanessa's research team found that women who viewed the "before" labiaplasty photos thought their labia were the smallest, followed by women who saw the post-labiaplasty pictures, followed by the women who saw pictures from a mainstream men's magazine.[13] So, what was happening? Is it possible that these women really had different sized labia? Probably not. We believe that they were using the pictures as reference points for what "normal" looks like and were judging the size of their inner labia based upon those judgments. In other words, the examples that we see of women's genitals may impact how we feel about our own.

Okay, so women thought their inner labia were bigger/smaller. Why is this interesting? To many it isn't—but considering you are reading a book about vulvas, we are going to assume that you are interested in the implications. First, this tells us that women's percep-tions of their labia size may be malleable. This also suggests that the media may play a role in how women perceive their genitals. This is no surprise given the media's reach in today's world; however, it is still interesting to note that our perceptions of something so important to some can be modified with just a few pictures. Finally, it is important because those women who perceive larger inner labia to be less attractive may find their own genitals less attractive if they believe that they are "larger" than their ideal.

VULVA MATCHING GAME

To make up for the fact that women and men are exposed to so few images of women's genital diversity, books that show images of women's vulvas (such as *Femalia*, *Petals*, and *I'll Show You Mine*) have helped to bridge this gap. Of course, as we all know from browsing photos of our friends and ourselves, people can look very different in one photo compared to another. The same is probably true for vulvas in that they may look different depending on the angle the photo is taken from, the lighting, or how a woman is sitting or standing or otherwise posed. We were delighted, then, when Catherine Johnson-Roehr, curator of The Kinsey Institute's art collection, showed us a remarkable series of images by institute photographer William Dellenback. Among the many things we like about this series is that there are multiple images taken for each woman, showing how different we can all look based on how we hold our labia or how we're sitting. What we hope this does for you is to show you how the same vulva on the same woman can vary so much. Not only is there genital diversity that can be celebrated for all of womankind but also for you as an individual.

Now for a fun little game: looking at the twelve images of vulvas from the institute's collection, see if you can identify which vulvas go together. We'll give you a hint: there are four women represented here and three images of each woman's vulva. Can you guess which vulvas belong to which women? (Answers are below the images—but don't peek.)

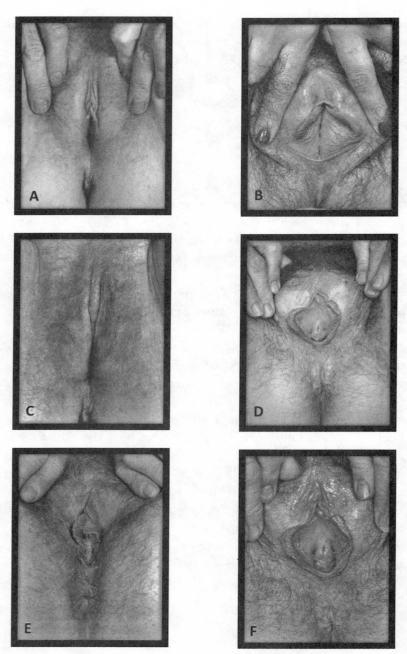

Answers: Woman 1 (J, G, E); Woman 2 (I, C, A); Woman 3 (D, F, L); Woman 4 (K, H, B)

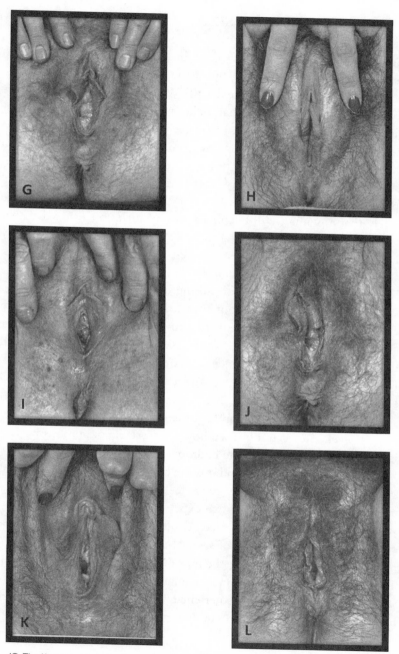

DOES SIZE MATTER?

Messages about penis size bombard us (check your "junk" or spam email folder if you disagree), but we rarely hear anything about the vulva. Is that because one size fits all? We wish. Unfortunately, there may be perceptions about what makes women's genitals more or less attractive. As with the penis, men's genital perceptions are out there for all to see and discuss, whereas women's genital concerns remain more hidden. Women may feel uncomfortable about their genital smell, size, or shape—though fortunately, most women don't feel persistently concerned or bothered about their genitals. It is more likely that a woman will become aware of such concerns when her genitals are relevant to the activity at hand. Does that mean any relevant activity? No—most women probably don't even think about their genitals much when they engage in day-to-day activities like going to the bathroom or pulling underwear on or off.

When do we think about them, then? Probably when we are concerned that someone else is thinking about them. When a lover goes down on her or a gynecologist asks a woman to scoot forward into the stirrups, she may suddenly become very aware of her genitals. Do I smell okay? How do I taste? What about my pubic hairstyle? Do I have too much pubic hair? Too little? Are my labia too long? Too short? These concerns crop up for different women at different times in their lives. They can influence how comfortable or anxious we feel in healthcare settings or in the bedroom.

It is often said that the mind is the biggest sex organ. Our mental state can influence how receptive we feel to being sexually touched or caressed, the ease with which we experience orgasm, or whether we want to have sex in the first place. Women may enjoy and/or experience orgasm from a variety of sexual activities including breast play, neck biting, and thigh licking; the list of non-genital activities goes on. That being said, for many women, genital stimulation is often a necessary element of their sexual experience. This includes everything from hand or finger stimulation to cunnilingus to vaginal intercourse and beyond. Some concerns may be temporary, while others are situation-dependent (e.g., When did I shower last? Have I shaved recently?), and others are somewhat more stable (e.g., Does my lover like my labia?). Any genital concerns have the potential to hinder women's enjoyment or pleasure. Whether it is a baby crying in the room, a telephone ringing by the side of the bed, or genital concerns badgering you inside your own head, it is tricky to stop and focus on pleasure with so much distraction.

In her dissertation research, Debby found that women's concerns about their genital appearance were more problematic than concerns about genital smell or taste when it came to whether or not a woman could sit back, relax, and enjoy receiving oral sex—or experience an orgasm from it. Vanessa and colleagues[14] also investigated the role of appearance-based concerns on women's sexual experience and found that women with concerns about their genital appearance reported significantly lower sexual self-esteem (feeling good about themselves in the bedroom), which translates into lower sexual satisfaction. It was even related to reduced intentions to use condoms or protective methods. This may be surprising at first, but it makes sense when you think about it. You are probably more likely to take care of those things that you love. In the same survey, the women were asked whether they enjoyed several sexual activities that involved their vulva. Whether or not they liked the various activities was probably dependent on many factors, but one commonly cited reason for their lack of enjoyment in the activities was their concerns about their genitals.

Despite popular conceptions that a woman's sexual complaints are due to her man's penis not being very long or her partner's technique, a woman's primary complaint is oftentimes actually about herself. Does that mean that there is nothing her lover can do to increase her sexual pleasure? Of course not. Psychological tips can be just as sexy as the physiological ones. When people ask us for one hint to enhance the quality of their sex lives, sometimes we tell them to simply remind their partners of how beautiful they are. This can be everything from her brain to her big brown eyes to her boobs or butt—just don't forget her lady bits. You can be perverted or polite about it—as long as you compliment her in a way that she's open to. Complimenting her vulva will open a dialogue in the bedroom that may make you both feel more at ease.

IS YOUR VULVA READY FOR ITS CLOSE-UP?

Hook-up Ready

Definition: The state of being physically and mentally prepared for a sexual encounter including the shaving of one's legs, genitals, etc.

Origin: A phrase that first made its appearance amongst drinks with a few girlfriends discussing an initial sexual encounter.

As properly used in the sentence: "I wanted to hook-up with him but couldn't because I wasn't hook-up ready," or "I snuck into his bathroom and dry-shaved with his razor because I wasn't hook-up ready." (Note: not recommended! (A) You should try to never share razors. It may increase the likelihood of STI transmission, and (B) Ouch! No one likes a dry shave, particularly not on your sensitive Sally.) Why are we filling you in on our cocktail party vernacular? Because we think that it nicely illustrates an interesting phenomenon. Some women may feel confident about their genitals regardless of the situation. Others may feel uncomfortable and in need of a little reassurance to get them revved up during the act, and still others are so shy, embarrassed, or ashamed about their genitals that they decide not to engage in sex that they otherwise want. These, of course, are not always three separate groups of women (although they certainly can be). For our friends, being hook-up ready is often only a state that they felt they needed to be in for their first sexual encounter with a new partner. It's kind of like avoiding sex because you're wearing unflattering granny panties and would rather wait until you feel like you're wearing sexier panties. But as time goes on, you feel comfortable breaking out your cotton day-of-the-week underwear.

In the same way that genital concerns may deter women from

seeking out sexual behavior that they may want, it may also prevent women from getting the healthcare that they need. Gynecologist Dr. Elizabeth Stewart, in her excellent book *The V Book*,[15] wrote about how women would often delay scheduling GYN exams so that they could have time to get their genitals ready (she urges women not to worry about how their genitals look or smell when it comes to healthcare). In another study, Debby found that women who felt more positively about their genitals were more likely to have had a recent gynecological exam. And in her dissertation work, Vanessa found that young women who are uncomfortable about the appearance of their genitals were more likely to be concerned that the exam would be embarrassing, making them feel anxious about the exam and eventually putting off a GYN exam entirely. This may have been

GETTING READY FOR THE GYN

One urban myth that we have heard refers to a woman who was rushing one day for her annual OB/GYN exam. She was in a hurry but wanted to make sure that she "washed up" before she saw the doctor. So, she grabbed one of her children's washcloths, wiped her vulva quickly, and took off to make her appointment on time. While at the doctor's office, everything went well; she didn't have to wait long and got a clean bill of health. However, she was puzzled by something the doctor had said during her examination. When she first got into the stirrups, the doctor mumbled, "fancy." She was a little disturbed by the comment but let it go in the hope that she had misheard. When she got home and went to the bathroom, she realized that she had not misheard at all. She had used her child's arts-and-crafts washcloth covered in glitter to wipe her genitals! She had presented the doctor with a special little surprise that day.

Take home point from the story: no matter how embarrassed you feel while visiting the gynecologist, just be thankful you are not covered in glitter (accidentally—more power to our sisters who intentionally go disco ball at the gynecologist!).

because some of these women were anticipating their first OB/GYN exam, so they had yet to receive any reassurance about their genitals (which they would *hopefully* get at the GYN). In a series of interviews with women after their exams, Drs. Oscarsson and Benzein[16] found that the only details that young women remembered after their first Pap smear was reassurance that their genitals were normal. Try to think back to your first exam. What can you remember?

THE CONTROVERSY OVER ELECTIVE GENITAL SURGERIES

In the UK, there is a popular show called *Embarrassing Bodies*.[17] The premise is an interesting one: men and women visit doctors to get a medical consult, treatment, and follow-up for a physical concern that may be considered, well, embarrassing. Many clips begin with patients talking about how their conditions have impacted their lives and how they have been too embarrassed to seek help in the past. (For some unknown reason, the patients find discussing and showing their "medical conditions" on camera to millions of viewers less distressing than bringing up the conversation in the privacy of their clinicians' offices, but we digress.)

The show is meant to normalize and de-stigmatize medical conditions. The TV show's web site (www.channel4embarrassingillnesses.com) features videos and information about what "normal vulvas" look like, how to perform a vulva self-exam, and other positive genital messages, which we applaud. Given that the TV show focuses on medical conditions that are supposed to be "embarrassing," it's perhaps not surprising that a number of women's complaints related to their genitals, a common site of taboo (even if we wish it weren't so). At least one video titled "Enlarged Labia" shows a woman's journey to the doctor's office to ask about her inner labia. After a quick consultation is done and shown on film (kudos to them for not hiding the genitals), the doctor delivers the good and bad news. She says, "Don't think that you are abnormal or a freak. What you have got is a normal variant. . . . I think that we could be able to help you with this. . . . I am not thinking gynecologist here, I am thinking more cosmetic surgeon."

We are not questioning the doctor's advice. The patient came in to see her with a concern, and the doctor told her that there was no reason to be concerned but if she was concerned, then there was a way to "fix" the problem. Is it possible that flipping through *Petals*, *Femalia*, or watching one of Betty Dodson's empowering films could have appeased the woman's concerns? Perhaps so, perhaps not. Regardless, we are not telling this story to question the doctor's approach to her patient. We are much more interested in how this consultation affected the viewers.

If you are a woman who has ever worried or wondered about the size of your labia, you likely would have watched closely as a woman receives a consult from a medical professional on this very topic. Sure, the doctor suggests that the appearance of the woman's labia is not abnormal, but she also suggests surgery in order to resolve the "problem." Meanwhile, the viewer is undoubtedly comparing her labia size with

A Guide to Common Female Genital Elective Surgeries

Procedure	Description	Reasons
Labiaplasty	Typically the reduction of the inner labia	Aesthetic concerns (length, symmetry, color); may reduce chafing during physical activity
Clitoral hood reduction ("clitoral unhooding")	Partial removal of the clitoral prepuce to expose the clitoral body	Thought to increase sexual stimulation/pleasure; aesthetic reasons
Perineoplasty or vaginoplasty ("vaginal rejuvenation")	Tightening of the vaginal canal; elevation/ strengthening of the perineal body	Increase sexual satisfaction/ partner's pleasure; assist with pelvic floor issues
Hymenoplasty	Alteration of the hymeneal ring	Gives the impression that the hymen is still intact; sexual reasons

Note: Read more about these surgeries in M. P. Goodman, "Female Cosmetic Genital Surgery," *Obstetrics and Gynecology* 113, no. 1, 154–59.

that of the woman onscreen to decipher whether she has a similar problem that would likely have a similar solution.

Embarrassing Bodies is far from the only show that has helped to popularize elective genital surgeries in the past decade. An increase in the number of television shows, newspaper articles, and web sites about elective genital surgeries has brought this subject to the public's attention. Try searching "large labia" (or even just "labia") on the Internet, and you will get a range of advertisements for labia-reduction surgery (called labiaplasty). Labiaplasty is designed to help women who suffer from labial hypertrophy. Sound scary? It isn't. That is just a medical term for long labia. How is it defined? It isn't; or at least it isn't defined very well. Some doctors have used two inches as a rough approximate guideline for classification.[18] Yet, just as a six-inch penis would look massive on some men and small on others, two-inch inner labia may appear longer on some women than they would on others. As such, many doctors use the patient's own feelings about and experiences with her labia to diagnose the patient. If a woman's labia present problems for the patient, the doctor may recommend surgical treatment as one possibility.

Why Labiaplasty?

Women may decide to get labiaplasty for many reasons. Of course, there are the aesthetic reasons, including concerns that labia are too long, too uneven, or too dark around the edges. There are also those women whose labia cause them physical discomfort (e.g., chafing or pain) while engaging in physical activities such as walking, biking, hiking, running, dancing, or horseback riding. One gynecologist we know who routinely performs genital surgeries told us that a large percentage of the women who request labiaplasty in his practice are women in the military because of the amount of physical activity required by their job (apparently the physical nature of their job results in labia discomfort for some women). This, of course, is anecdotal. There is very little research on who gets these surgeries, why they get them, and how they feel about them. We are doing our best to remedy this with a study we currently have underway with a surgeon who specializes in these procedures. The data are still being collected, so be on the lookout for the results.

I have not seriously considered labiaplasty but I have on more than one occasion declared it the cosmetic surgery I would have if I were ever to have cosmetic surgery. I am confident and comfortable, appearance-wise with my genitals. I love the way my partner can pull and suck at my inner labia. I even like the way they look jutting out between my outer labia when closed. BUT—they can be hazardous! They get pinched in lace underwear, jeans, tight pants, hose . . . anything! This can happen in the most unfortunate instances and is excruciating until manually adjusted—not always possible in polite company. So—I get the controversy that surrounds labiaplasty and I am always sad to hear women talk about the embarrassment they feel around their large labia minora, but the very real physical discomfort and occasional pain is not often validated.

—STEPHANIE, 25, Canada

Elective genital surgeries such as labiaplasty have been the subject of a great deal of controversy within the scientific and medical communities. In a discussion on this topic at an international medical conference, a gynecologist from France indicated that she sometimes performs labiaplasty for women who are sexually bothered or distressed by their labia size or appearance. Some of the American gynecologists took issue with her statement, with a couple saying that they only perform labiaplasty for patients if their labia get in the way of daily activities such as exercise and going to the gym. This interested Debby, who joined the conversation by asking why being comfortable exercising is any more important than being comfortable having sex. After all, if a woman feels that her labia get in the way of her sex life—if she's embarrassed about them in spite of being well aware that others consider them normal or beautiful, or if her labia are uncomfortably pushed inside her vagina during intercourse, then why should she be turned down for surgery?

As sex researchers and educators, we don't believe that one activity (sex or exercise) should be prioritized over the other. As long as a woman is fully informed about all other options (some women may just need to flip through a book of realistic vulva images) and is choosing surgery for herself (some women report being pressured by their partner), then what is offered to one woman should be offered to all. And this is coming from two women who adore vulvas and vaginas and who wish, from their hearts, that every woman could feel happy with their genitals (and their breasts, thighs, freckles, and hair) as they are, rather than feel a need for surgery.

The only time I have ever felt ashamed or really less-than-satisfied with my genitals was my mother-in-law's fault. She's got some weird, creepy competition thing going on with me, and since I first got pregnant has made it a point to tell me, my friends, random waiters, that HER vagina is as tight as it ever was because SHE had a C-section. Then, in the delivery room immediately after I'd given vaginal birth to my first daughter and was having the episiotomy stitched up, she told my midwife to "put in an extra stitch for my son— or maybe two; that looks like he'll be throwing a hot dog down a hallway." There's nothing like having your husband's mother standing there looking at your stretched and bruised and bleeding genitals and cheerily declaring them to be no longer fit for her son to fuck to really make you wish you'd gone with the Fentanyl instead of the epidural. I just keep reminding myself that she was taught anatomy by nuns, it's not all her fault she's completely retarded about how lady parts work.

—GLORIA, 32, Kansas

Being offered the surgery and going through with the surgery are two different things. Insurance companies tend not to cover such surgeries,[19] meaning that these procedures often cost several thousand dollars. In addition to money, they require a small amount of time for the surgery and a larger amount of time to recover from the surgery (often several weeks to a couple months). There is not a great deal of good research on how painful these procedures are but like any major surgery, we imagine, and have heard from some patients, that there is likely a fair amount of potential for pain or discomfort.[20]

The controversy about elective genital surgeries is not only about who should be allowed to get elective cosmetic surgery; some genital advocates are critical about the way that these surgeries are marketed to women. In addition to labiaplasty, other elective genital surgeries include those intended to resize and reshape the clitoral hood, tighten the vaginal canal (vaginal "rejuvenation"), and surgery to reduce the size of the mons pubis. There are also procedures designed to create a fake hymen to partially cover a woman's vaginal entrance. Most of these surgeries have not been well researched (we're trying to change this in conjunction with an OB/GYN we know who performs such surgeries).

Some feminist scholars, among others, are well-known critics of labiaplasty, suggesting that it pathologizes the diversity of women's genitals.[20-23] This means that the existence and marketing of the surgery creates the perception that there is only one "normal" vulva appearance and that any other appearance outside of this single appearance norm is viewed as abnormal and in need of fixing. This idea is further perpetuated by web sites that show "before" and "after" pictures, which can be used to define and differentiate between appropriate and abnormal vulva appearances. It is a complicated issue without a simple solution. What do you think? Should all women have access to these surgeries? And how should they be presented to women so that they can best make such an important decision?

WHAT'S THE (I)DEAL?

Have you ever stopped to wonder where breast augmentation procedures came from? At what point was it decided that having a D cup was preferable to a B? What about waist and hip sizes? There are evolutionary and social explanations offered for all of these ideals. Evolutionary theorists suggest that these ideals may be markers of youth and fertility, while feminist social constructionists point to the ways in which these ideals have helped to maintain a patriarchal society. Female genital ideals are the new kid on the block. Sure, we don't know a lot about her, but that has not stopped everyone from wondering, where did she come from?

Before we go any further, let's take a step back and think about what the genital-appearance ideal is (if there is one). If our analysis of mainstream men's magazines is correct, it means the ideal vulva will have no pubic hair, a petite clitoris, and practically invisible inner labia. Sound familiar? If you have ever changed a baby girl's diaper, her vulva may look a lot like this. As women, we are told that there will be a lot of changes that will happen to our bodies as we hit puberty. We will develop breasts, experience a widening of our hips, start menstruating, and even sprout some hair down there. Yet no one really talks about the fact that our inner labia and clitoris also may grow during puberty.[24] This is why vulvas may look more similar prior to puberty but show such enormous diversity following puberty. What does this have to do

---

ALL OVER THE MAP

Beach season can be an anxiety-provoking time for many women. For some women in the United States, it signifies a time of intense workouts and heavy spray-tanning. However, these beauty ideals are not one-size-fits-all. In Southeast Asia, many beauty creams come with skin lightener because fairer skin is perceived to be a sign of beauty.[25] In certain parts of western Africa, you can forget the Western stick-figure body ideal. For them, heavier women are perceived as most beautiful.[25] Thus, it makes sense that vulva-appearance ideals would also vary cross-culturally. In Japan, women with large labia are called "winged butterflies" and are considered a "sexual delicacy."[26] In certain parts of central Africa, it is a custom for women to stretch their inner labia because it is perceived as more beautiful and likely to increase sexual satisfaction. Some classify this practice as female genital mutilation, though this is highly contestable.

with the "vulva ideal," you ask? Perhaps nothing, but both evolutionary theorists and social constructionists believe that women's youth is valued either as a marker of fertility or of innocence/dependence. Society's value on women's innocence/dependence is just one of several possible explanations for this ideal. What do you think the reason is?

TWAT TO DO IF . . .

You are a healthcare provider giving a genital exam.

    This is a question we get time and time again: How do we help our patients feel better about their genitals? If your first reaction is to compliment your patient's genitals, better think again. You wouldn't tell your patient she has a nice rack, and it is probably best to extend that policy downstairs. According to one research study, women were not very fond of being complimented on the appearance of their genitals.[27] Instead, consider saying something like, "your genitals look perfectly normal" or "healthy." Better yet, Nick and Sayaka Karras, the authors of *Petals*, are working on an amazing new project. They created beautiful posters with a variety of diverse vulva images (sepia-toned or color images are available) with the saying, "Each Beautiful, and as Unique as a Snowflake," underneath the images (www.ilovemypetals.com). Nick and Sayaka Karras made these posters in the hope that doctors (and educators and others) would hang them in their offices or other relevant places so that women could see how normal their genitals actually are. As the famous saying goes, a picture is worth a thousand words.

You love someone who has genital concerns.

    Scientists don't know much about what men think about women's genitals. Rhonda Reinholtz and Charlene Muehlenhard conducted one study at the University of Kansas.[28] They asked a few hundred college students to complete a questionnaire on their thoughts and feelings about one another's genitals. The male participants reported feeling more positively about both their own genitals and their female partners' genitals than the female participants reported feeling about male or female genitals. In another study that Debby conducted, she also found that men generally felt more positively about women's genitals than women themselves did. In particular, the majority of men indicated that they enjoyed performing oral sex (something the women who completed the survey indicated they worry about).

We are also vulva advocates, which means that we talk to people about genitals fairly often. To be fair, this means that the men in our lives may be lying out of fear that we will shake our heads in disappointment if they slander women's genitals. Nevertheless, from our research experience, many men love that women's genitals come in all shapes, sizes, and colors.

You are a genital advocate.

Sometimes this means just being a positive reinforcement to a friend who has concerns. Maybe it means organizing a genital advocacy event for a group of (girl)friends (see this chapter's craft idea for one possible suggestion). Perhaps it is as simple as reading this book in a public place, such as a subway, park bench, or coffee shop, so that others can get a glimpse of the place vulvas should have in the world. We feel very fortunate to have so many opportunities to spread genital pride. Being educators at a university puts us in a particularly good place to open up discussions about thoughts and feelings about genitals. Debby has taught over fifteen semesters' worth of human sexuality courses to thousands of students. We both like to start our genital lectures in similar ways: having the students write or shout out every word that they can think of for male and female genitals. It can be difficult to talk about something that you feel funny saying, so we get it all out in the open in the beginning. We remind our students that anything goes and listen as they laugh and giggle when they realize that they are able to say "cunt" and "pussy" in a classroom without getting in trouble. Once we have talked about the language around women's genitals, we are ready to begin our discussion.

Last fall, Vanessa was involved in a genital advocacy conference where she was asked by the planner, Dr. Leonore Tiefer, to show a series of vulva diversity videos and tape the students' reactions. It was supposed to be an "intervention" that any college professor could do regardless of his or her background. Vanessa went to about five different college classrooms and showed the students two videos. The first video was a documentary about the making of the book *Petals*.[11] It focused primarily on the psychological impact of modeling for and viewing the photos. The video also concentrates on some of the serious concerns and issues that women may struggle with when relating to their vulvas, and it is a very powerful film. The next film is a more light-hearted look at the vulva. Betty Dodson's *Viva la Vulva* takes viewers through a masturbation circle, starting with a genital show-and-tell with many different women's vulvas on display. All vulvas are applauded as Betty uses words like "baroque" and "sunset" to describe their vulva shapes and colors. Did it make a difference? Sure, there were one or two students who were not fans, but we are hopeful that the experience was positive for most; certainly, many of the students expressed their reactions in thoughtful and insightful ways. Although we are very thankful to have "official" educator titles that allow us to show these types of films, "educators" can take many forms, as a mother, daughter, sister, brother, friend, or lover. So don't be afraid to share the vulva love!

TEST YOUR VQ

1. How has the portrayal of pubic hair patterns changed over the past twenty years?
   a. Pubic hair patterns are relatively similar.
   b. Pubic hair is now presented as slightly more abundant than it was twenty years ago.
   c. It is slightly less common to present pubic hair now than it was twenty years ago.
   d. Twenty years ago, representations of women in magazines were approximately 90 percent more likely to have pubic hair.

2. If you have ever wondered whether your genital appearance is normal,
   a. you might find it helpful to talk to a sex-positive, vulva-positive healthcare provider (chances are, you're "normal")
   b. there is probably something wrong with your genitals
   c. you should Google it
   d. you should talk to a plastic surgeon

3. If you want to be a genital advocate, you should consider
   a. promoting positive messages in response to negative genital comments on the Internet
   b. throwing a genital craft party
   c. joining us on Facebook or following us on Twitter
   d. all of the above

Answers

   1. d
   2. a
   3. d

Spraying, Dyeing, and Douching . . . Oh My!

*W*hen did women's genitals get their own aisle?" we wondered aloud recently during a trip to our local drugstore. Don't get us wrong; we are all about genital awareness. We just couldn't remember when the market had expanded from pads and tampons to include everything from dyes to douches. Are these products really necessary? More importantly, are they really safe? In this chapter, we'll give you the lowdown on all those products marketed for your downtown.

PERIOD PRODUCT PARTICULARS

Love her or hate her, your dear Aunt Flo decides to stop in for another visit. Sometimes she phones ahead to let you know she'll be coming to (down)town; other times, she may just surprise you. Prepared or not, there she is, on your doorstep. Time to make some decisions about where she is going to stay. Fortunately, you have a lot of options—and they've gotten better over time, so even if you've been in the period game for decades, listen up.

The most popular period products are tampons and pads. Some women choose to use only one, others use both at the same time, while some women believe that there is a time and place for both. Dr. Czerwinski conducted a survey of over seven hundred women in California about their use of various feminine products and found that similar percentages of women reported using pads and tampons with approximately half of the women reporting that they use both.[1]

PAD DOWN

The pad is a product with many names including (but not limited to) maxi pad, menstrual pad, sanitary pad, sanitary towel, and sanitary napkin; for simplicity's sake, we are going to refer to it simply as a pad. Thinner versions of pads are often called pantyliners and may be worn on days with a lighter menstrual flow.

As a child I was told my genitals were nasty and disgusting. As a young girl going through puberty I had to come to grips with my identity and my genitals. I have a wonderful well functioning body part. My monthly cycles made it hard at first to overcome the dirty and disgusting message. Over time and education about the function and purpose of my body I came to love and enjoy being a woman.

—Caroline, 35, Utah

If you are like many women, the first thing that probably comes to mind when thinking of pads is pink cardboard boxes with individually wrapped plastic packages containing "cotton" pads (that often have a plastic covering) that come complete with an adhesive strip. This is a description of the contemporary pad on today's market, but they have taken many forms throughout history, dating back to the fourth century.

Pads were originally made from an assortment of absorbent materials. Disposable pads are a somewhat more recent phenomenon with the first pads requiring a belt/band typically worn around the waist to stay in place. We've never tried one, but we have heard that there was a lot of twisting, shifting, and sliding. The invention of pads with adhesive backs made the pad somewhat more comfortable and convenient. However, even those earliest disposable/stickable pads (which we have used) had their flaws. It was difficult to get through a few hours of menstruation without dyeing the sides of your panties a shade of menstrual red/brown (which is surprisingly still not a Crayola color or paint shade in the Martha Stewart Living paint palette).

The Wind Beneath Our Wings

The development of "wings" not only gave the pads a snazzy paper-airplane look, they also helped them stay in place and kept the blood from crossing over to the other side. We were fans. Then there was the somewhat recent invention of pads for thongs. We know that thongs are not for everyone (perhaps especially true for women with genital pain), but it is nice to have a pad option for all panty choices. Some women like these pads because they stay "close to your body," while others think they are too thin or that wearing a padded thong defeats the purpose of a thong all together. We say, to each their own!

As with silverware, plates, and diapers, having a pad that is disposable makes life more convenient. You can pull it off and toss it in those special little trashcans strategically placed in public bathrooms. Toss them and forget them, right? Sure, but the pad's story doesn't end when you throw it away. In fact, that pad's story is never-ending (at least not in your lifetime). Most pads are made from polypropylene, which is non-biodegradable (this is why we put cotton in quotes earlier in the chapter). If you use pads, take a second and think about how many pads you go through in one day. Let's say you use one at night and change it about every four hours while awake. That adds up to about five pads a day. Five pads a day for five days is twenty-five pads, which adds up to somewhere around three hundred pads over twelve months! Doesn't sound like a lot? Try finding a place to stack three hundred pads in your home. Now does it sound like a lot?

Turning Your "Red" Days "Green"

If creating this much period-product waste concerns you, there are other options available. There are disposable pads that claim to be biodegradable. They are not widely available but may be found in health-food stores or similar locations. Even if you are not concerned with the environmental impact of pads, you may want to consider the impact on something else: your wallet. Depending on the price of each pad, costs can add up quickly!

How can you save money and the environment? Consider making your own pad. There are even underwear with pads already in them so that they don't scrunch and bunch (see Resources). Just toss them in with the rest of your wash (pre-wash if heavily soaked), and they are ready to go for round two.

TAMP-ON-IT

Perhaps, like many women, you have a memory like this one:

It was a hot summer day and the pool beckoned. All of your friends were having fun, splashing and enjoying the crisp, cool blue water. You wanted to splash around, too, rather than sit on the lounge chair or your towel alone, but you had your period, and you had only been using pads up to this point.

It was time to make a choice. You could

a. stay inside by your lonesome.
b. swelter in the heat, pretending that you just felt like "dipping your feet in."
c. stick a pad to the bottom of your bathing suit (although those images of babies with droopy diapers were a definite deterrent).
d. hope the old wives tale that people do not menstruate in the water is actually true.
e. tamp-on-it.

Some women start using tampons during their very first period and others never decide to use tampons. On the other hand, many women transition from pads to tampon use. There are many different

V-CRAFT: HOW TO MAKE A NO-SEW COOCHIE CARRYING CLUTCH

You are sitting at a meeting or in class when it happens. To your horror, your tampon has over-expanded and is slowly slipping out of your vaginal comfort zone, or you suddenly feel a surge of menstrual blood that may or may not have slipped past the defense. Time to take your tampon out!

You need to sneak off to the bathroom, but you also need to be prepared, and your protection is currently stashed away between books and papers. You go on a hunt and find your treasure. Now what? If you don't have pockets you may find yourself in a conundrum. You can proudly parade across the room with your tampon/pad in hand or lug your giant purse/backpack/briefcase across the room. Then, after you finally manage to smuggle your tampon/pad into the bathroom—you notice it! That's right—it's happened to all of us: pencil shavings/dirt/food crumbs have managed to find their way to your tampon/pad, and now they are stuck to the wrapper.

This is a situation that we can all probably relate to in one way or another. Fortunately, we have a craft solution: a no-sew coochie carrying case! Design it to look like a vulva to make a bold statement, or use your favorite fabrics for a more concealed one.

What You Will Need

- A favorite fabric. Pick one that you love, but try to steer clear of fabrics with stretch. If you are making a coochie carrying case, you will need two different fabrics to differentiate between the outer and inner labia. We recommend a material with some movement for the inner labia. Silk (or imitation) is always a good bet.
- Masking/duct tape. Most masking tape comes in a shade of brown. If you like this, great! If not, keep shopping around. You may be able to find colored masking tape at your local hardware store or through the Internet. If you are unable to find colored masking tape, clear masking tape will allow your fabric to shine through.

- Double-sided tape (optional for pubic hair)
- Cotton if you want to give your inner labia a little puff. The kind sold at the grocery/drug store in the nail-polish remover section should be just fine (optional for inner labia stuffing).
- A ruler for measuring the fabric
- A pencil for marking the fabric
- A stapler. It doesn't have to be super fancy, but it should be able to staple through a few pieces of paper relatively easily.
- Something to close up the bag. Velcro is the easiest, but zippers are more likely to impress your friends. A pipe cleaner is definitely the least-expensive option and probably the best if you are providing supplies for lots of people or creating more than one carrying case (optional).
- Hair. We don't recommend using your own (although you can by cutting and taping the ends to a piece of paper. Your local craft store should carry some relatively inexpensive doll wigs that should work). If not, your Halloween/costume store is sure to have a wig that should do the "trick" (get it—because it's Halloween) (optional).

What to Do

Outer Labia

1. Let's start by cutting the fabric that you want to use for the outside of the bag. The length is entirely up to you. Are you just using this for tampons/pads, or do you want to use it for other things as well? If tampons and pads, are they large or are they small? How many do you want to carry at one time? Take all of these things into consideration when deciding on the size. Somewhere between six and twelve inches is typical. Measure approximately ½ inch from the top of the fabric and ½ inch from the right side of the edge of the fabric and mark those spots. Now, draw a rectangle or square to your desired size, starting at the ¾ inch and ½ inch marks. Now draw another line ½ inch from the left-hand side of the square/rectangle. You are going to cut along the line that you just drew so that you have three sides of the square/rectangle cut out. Fold the material over so

that it is doubled on top of the fabric and trace the outline of the material. You are now going to cut out the remainder of the square. So when you are finished, it should be one long piece of material, with both sides of the box or rectangle connected at the center.

2. It's taping time! Get out your masking tape and cover one entire side of the fabric with masking tape. You are obviously going to want to cover the side of the fabric that you don't want to be visible on the inside of the bag.

Inner Labia

1. Now you are going to cut the inner labia (labiaplasty reference not intended). The inner labia are going to be the same width as the outer labia but a little bit shorter in length (about ½ inch). To start, measure out a square/rectangle about the same length as the material that you just cut for the outer labia and deduct about ½ inch from the top. Mark that rectangle/square with your pencil. Now create three more boxes connected to the original box you just created (it should look like one giant box or rectangle). Cut along the outside of the box/rectangle.

2. You should now be ready to create the inner labia. Fold the material in half once, length-wise, so that you have a long tube (without an enclosed bottom). If the material has two sides, fold the material so that the "bad" side is folded on the inside and the side that you want is facing you.

3. Stuffing time! Take the cotton balls and pull them slightly so that they are less ball-shaped (this will give you lumpy inner labia) and more fluffy and long. Once you have a handful, place them along the inside of the tube. Keep going until the tube has a little fluff to it. Be careful not to overfill. If too full, there won't be room for anything else besides the coochie inside of your clutch!

Clutch Handle

Set aside the inner labia for now. It is time to create the handle for the clutch. Cut a piece of fabric about two inches thick and a foot and a half long. Follow the same instructions as you did for the inner labia (minus the stuffing). As a reminder: place the ugly-fabric side out, duct-tape the bottom of the fabric and staple to make sure it stays in place. Now flip it inside out so that the staples and duct tape are on the inside of the strap. Set it aside—we'll come back to it later.

Pubic Hair
Cut a strip of double-sided tape the length of the outer labia fabric (the first fabric that you cut). Tape the end to the edge of a table or flat surface with a ledge. Now, if you are using a wig, it's time to give it a haircut! Trim the hair to the length that you want to keep the pubic hair (a half-inch to an inch works best). Now carefully tape the ends of the pubic hair to the edge of the duct tape so that the hair takes up no more than half of the tape. Set aside and try not to disrupt. We will come back to it in just a minute.

And It All Comes Together

Okay, almost there! This is the tricky part. We are going to put all the pieces together. Start by laying out the outer labia (or bag fabric) so that the duct tape is on the outside facing you.

1. Attach the inner labia: Surgery time! We are going to attach the inner labia to the outer labia fabric. Lay the inner labia on top of the outer labia so that the open edge of the inner labia meets the edge of the outer labia fabric. Duct-tape the end of the fabric together so that the duct tape wraps from the inside of the inner-labia fabric to the non-duct taped side of the outer-labia fabric.

2. Put some hair on there: Fold over the top of the outer labia approximately ¼ inch. Take the tape off of the ledge and place it on top of the folded-over fabric so that pubic hair is on top and the back side of the tape with pubic hair is on top of the flap.

Wrap the other half of the tape around the other side of the flap to hold it in place. Press down.

3. Attach the bag closer/pipe cleaner: Now we are going to put in the pipe cleaner so that we can open and close the bag. Simply slip the pipe cleaner in the tube that you just created. If your pipe cleaner is too short, you can twist the ends of two pieces together. If it is too long, simply cut it. Staple the edge of the pipe cleaner to the edge of the outer fabric. Try to get as close to the end as possible. Now fold over the top edge of the outer labia about ½ inch. Place a piece of duct tape over the top of the pubic hair tape. If you can, try to keep a straight line because this will stay visible on the inside of the bag. Do not tape over the ends of the tube.

4. Attach the clutch strap: Slip the clutch strap inside the open pocket that you just created when you duct-taped the tube together with pipe cleaner/pubic hair. Put in a single staple.

5. It all comes together: Fold the fabric widthwise once so that it is approximately the size of the clutch. Fold so that the duct tape, pubic hair, and inner labia are all visible. Wrap the clutch handle back around so that it is facing the inside material (not duct-tape covered) of the bag. Now put staples around two of the four edges. You may want to do two rows for extra security. Do not staple the top with the pipe cleaner/pubic hair or the edge that was naturally created when you folded the fabric. Now tape over the edges that you stapled with duct tape.

6. That's so clutch! Time to flip it inside out to see your creative new coochie clutch! Carefully invert the materials so that the inner labia and duct tape are now on the inside of the bag. Violà! You have coochie clutch complete with a strap, inner labia pocket, and fun pubic hair trim. No more hanging your head in shame as you head to the bathroom with your tampons/pads. You can stride with your new clutch in (your own) style.

reasons why women may do this. Wanting to go swimming is one of them. Other times, girls who take dance classes find that wearing a pad feels uncomfortable or awkward when they're wearing leotards and tights. Or they tire of staining the sides of their panties, wings or no wings.

Oftentimes, people have questions about tampons. We are not sure why there are so many myths about them, but we are happy that people are being inquisitive about what's going on inside their bodies. If you have mastered the period waters for years, you may have forgotten some of these common questions or myths from your childhood or adolescence. If you're a mom, aunt, or teacher, you may find it helpful to look through these questions and myths so that you can best support the young girls in your life. When Debby has been invited to speak with fifth- and sixth-grade girls about puberty, she has often fielded similar kinds of questions—questions that she and her friends had years earlier—reminding us that the more things change, the more they stay the same.

Here are some of the most frequently asked questions we hear about tampons:

At what age is it appropriate to start using a tampon?

There is no right or wrong age. There isn't even a right or wrong stage of development. As we said, some women choose to use tampons during their first period, while others never use them. The right time to use a tampon is when and if you decide you want to. If you start using tampons and then decide you want to stop, that's okay too.

Are women who use tampons no longer virgins?

Most people define virginity based on whether or not they have had "sex" with another person. In that sense, if you have not had sexual intercourse or penetration with a partner, then you are still a virgin whether you have used no tampons, one tampon, or five thousand tampons over the course of your life.

Of course, "sex" can be defined in many ways, but we have not met many people who define it as tampon insertion. That being said, we recognize and respect that people may define different terms in diverse ways. For some people, virginity means never having had vaginal intercourse. For others, it means never having had any kind of sex, such as vaginal sex, anal sex, or oral sex. And for other people, virginity may mean having an intact hymen. Even if you don't believe this, you may have wondered: Is there any validity to the suggestion that those women who have used tampons cannot be virgins? Several researchers at Children's Hospital and Harvard Medical School were apparently curious as well.[2] They included three hundred young women in a study investigating this question. The young women were split evenly into three groups based on their previous experiences: Group 1 reported that they had never had sexual intercourse and only used pads during their periods; Group 2 also reported that they had never had sexual intercourse but used tampons; and Group 3 reported that they had sexual intercourse in the past. The researchers found that the hymen differed for those women who had a history of sexual intercourse and those who did not. Conversely, there were no significant differences between the groups of women who did or did not use tampons. They did find a difference in something less expected: the participants' perceptions of their speculum examinations. Only about a quarter of the pad-using participants in Group 1 felt that the exam was easy as compared to over half of the young women who reported using tampons.

To summarize, tampon use doesn't "de-virginize" a woman, and it doesn't make her hymen look different from those of women who don't use tampons. Tampon use may, however, help women to become more comfortable with vaginal penetration and thus more comfortable with gynecological exam procedures, such as a speculum examination.

Because of the lack of skill building around tampons (and other period devices), I was very uncertain how to work with my genitals for a long time. There should be more of this information given and skills worked on early on, so people don't get negative impressions of their genitals through these things. They definitely had a negative impact on me, until I met a sexual partner who was much more positive.

—MERCEDES, 28, New York

How do I insert a tampon?

Every woman probably has a slightly different method for inserting a tampon. Some lift a leg, others prefer squatting, and others just stay right where they are sitting. The best method will be the one that works best for you. Inserting a tampon is very different based upon whether you use tampons with or without applicators (see the following section, "Choosing a Tampon That's Right for You").

If you use a tampon with an applicator, resist the urge to pull apart the pieces when you open up the package. The tampon stays in the top component and is pushed through by the bottom portion. If you use a non-applicator tampon, try to press your fingertip against the bottom of the tampon, where the string is (not all the way—just enough to be able to push it) and push it in. It may take a few tries, but you'll get it.

How do I know when a tampon is in right?

Women commonly say that they know they have a tampon in far enough when they can no longer feel it inside of them. If you are having a difficult time with it, don't be too hard on yourself. Every woman and every tampon is a little different, so don't be afraid to give something new a try!

Can my tampon get lost inside of my body?

The good news is that your vagina is not like the pipes in your house. You cannot get something lost in it, and you don't need to get it "snaked" if there is something stuck in it. The vagina ends at the very small cervix and a tampon cannot get through the cervix. So no, your vagina is not a black hole in which things can get lost forever, and no tampon (or any other reasonably sized object) will get lost inside it.

What happens if I forget that I have a tampon in and leave it for too long—like, for several days?

Although tampons can't get "lost" inside the vagina (it's not that big and it ends at the cervix), it is true that some women forget to remove a tampon and may leave it in for days. This is not a good idea, but it happens sometimes. Maybe your mind is elsewhere when switching tampons and you insert a new tampon before remembering to take out the first one. Or maybe in the heat of the moment, you forget to take it out before having sex. Or maybe you just forgot it was in there at the end of your period and went on with life, until one day things felt or smelled funny, and you stuck your finger in your vagina to check things out. These things happen. If it happens to you, don't panic. Start by trying to get the tampon out. The string may have gotten lost but that just means that you are going to have to insert your fingers into your vagina and, as we say, "go fishing for it." Before embarking on the excavation, start by washing your hands thoroughly. It also can't hurt to give your fingernails a quick look to make sure there are no sharp edges (file them down if needed).

Forgotten tampons usually come out without a hitch. But in case it doesn't, here are some tips. You may find that it helps to try a few different positions to get the right angle. You may feel more comfortable lying down with pillows to prop you up, standing with one foot on the counter or squatting. Using a bit of water-based lubricant on your finger or around your vaginal opening can ease the process. If you have the benefit of a partner or open-minded friend around, it may help to enlist his/her help. If you feel nervous about it, you may want to offer him/ her a pair of gloves (latex gloves or similar—not winter gloves!). If neither you nor your friend/lover/open-minded someone is able to find it, do not assume that the problem has mysteriously resolved itself. Try to get into your gynecologist's office as soon as you can. Don't be embarrassed! Many gynecologists have told us that they see this kind of thing all the time. People have lost far more unusual things inside their vaginas.

In order to avoid having this happen to you, we recommend practicing inserting a finger inside your vagina. It only takes a second to do, and if you get in the habit of doing it every now and then—and most definitely in the days following your period—then you will be far more likely to catch a stray tampon if you forgot you had one up there. If there's ever a good reason to become more comfortable touching your vagina, this is it!

When I was in 8th grade, I didn't know what the word "pussy" meant. This boy in my class started bothering me about it asking me to tell him what it meant. I lied and said I did know, which just made him egg me on all the more. When it was clear by my face that I had no idea what I was talking about, he said "You idiot. You don't even know what you have." Then he told his friends. I inferred what pussy meant and was so humiliated. This doesn't necessarily have to do with my physical perceptions of my genitals, but his mean, caustic attitude towards me and my genitals filled me with shame, which extended into my emotional feelings about my genitals. It took a long time to get over.

—Amber, 23, California

What's the deal with TSS?

TSS stands for toxic shock syndrome, a scary name that has likely sent fear into the hearts and vaginas of many tampon users over the years. The truth of the matter is it is very rarely associated with tampon use. You can read more about TSS in Chapter 2: A Healthy, Happy Vulva.

CHOOSING A TAMPON THAT'S RIGHT FOR YOU

Just as women have options to choose from in terms of shoe styles, condom features, and phones, there are various options to choose from when it comes to tampons, too.

Size

Most tampons, regardless of the brand, will come in several different sizes. Don't worry; this is not like your shoe size, so there is no need for measurements. Some women have a difficult time inserting a large tampon and other women have a tricky time keeping in a smaller one. However, for most, tampons are one-size-fits-all.

Instead of choosing a tampon for comfort, women will often pick their tampons based on their menstrual flow. While some women always have heavier periods, other's menstrual flow never seems like more than a trickle. For women with a heavier flow, the choice is relatively clear: bigger tampons are often more absorbent. For many women, their flow will start heavier and slow down as the days progress. For these women, there are mixed packages. A relatively recent invention, we were super excited to see these in our regular tampon line-up available in many drugstores. The packages we've seen will give you approximately equal numbers of three different tampon absorbencies to "go with the flow." Although some women find that they run out of one type before the others, it is still a great idea. They are also good for women who are new to tampons and not really sure which size is best for them. Don't be afraid to try them out and find the fit that is best for you!

Shape and Materials

There is not much variability in the materials used for tampons. They are typically made from rayon and/or cotton, and organic tampons are normally made from 100 percent organic cotton without the bleach used on other tampons. One of the most important ways that tampons differ is in the way they extend as they absorb.

Some tampons will extend lengthwise, while others extend radially (width-wise). The ones that extend radially tend to have little grooves in the sides. Each method has its advantages/disadvantages.

Tampons that extend lengthwise can start to "pop out" if you leave them in for too long (sounds a little like a pop-up turkey thermometer). This can be a little uncomfortable if you are not in a place where you can change it. The radial ones, on the other hand, can start to make you feel uncomfortable as well, but it may be a little less obvious. Some find that they get slight stomachaches when they leave these tampons in for too long. So, while neither one is ideal, both work great. It is just a matter of which is the least distracting/uncomfortable for you!

Applicator

If you ask most women to divide tampons into two groups, many will differentiate them based on whether or not they have an applicator. An applicator can come in many different materials (e.g., cardboard, plastic) and essentially includes a smaller tub inside of a larger one. The tampon sits inside of the larger tube and is pushed out when you press on the smaller tube. Some women like an applicator because it prevents you from having (or "getting," depending on your point of view) to insert the tampon into your vagina. Non-applicator users are often very committed to their cause. It is not only better for the environment; some women simply prefer the "fit" or the convenience of being able to carry smaller tampons around in their purses.

Recently, the primary non-applicator tampon brand, o.b., disappeared from many store shelves across America. For many women, it was a catastrophe and was dubbed by some in the media as the "Tamponcalypse." According to the manufacturer, there was simply a pause in the shipping, which caused the problem, and they promised that they would be back out soon. This did little to reassure fans who panicked when they couldn't find their treasured tampon. They quickly became a black-market item, with women paying in excess of $100 for a few boxes found online. When o.b. tampons started to slowly appear on shelves again, women were overjoyed and united to find a place to purchase them. There was even an online treasure map for women to mark where they were able to find the tampons once they came back on the market. Sound like commitment? Well, that's nothing. In the midst of the Tamponcalypse, we happened across a lonely o.b. sitting on the sidewalk while walking back from lunch one day. At first, we wondered if this was perhaps one of those jokes that little tricksters play, where they drop a valuable item on the floor and then pull it away or glue it to the ground for giggles as the poor sap tries to pry it off the floor. It felt like finding a $20 bill on the ground. After staring at it for some time and trying to justify the fact that it *was* still wrapped in plastic and thus likely clean inside, we decided to walk away and leave it on the ground. Would the story have been different if we both had not already stocked up at home? If we thought it was the only o.b. left on the planet? Would we have fought each other over it? Perhaps. However, the alternative ending to the story would have been less likely to find its way into the book. I mean, who wants to tell the world that you've picked up a tampon off the ground and may use it later on in the month?

MENSTRUAL CUPS AND SPONGES

This section would not be complete without discussing some of the other options on the market: notably, menstrual cups. As with pads, your use of tampons may have you feeling concerned about the impact on the environment (particularly if you use plastic applicators) and/or the cost of frequent tampon use. If so, consider using menstrual cups.

There are several brands of menstrual cups including the Keeper, the Moon Cup, and the DivaCup. Although the idea of a tampon alternative may sound new and novel, they have actually been around since the 1930s. Shaped like plastic (technically silicone) bells, the bell end is folded twice and inserted into your vagina. As with a bell, there is a stem at the top that can be used for pulling the menstrual cup out when you are ready to change it. The menstrual cup holds approximately an ounce of liquid, so it is good for both heavy and light days. To change it, just pull it out, empty it and wash or wipe it off. Ready to reinsert! They are supposed to last upwards of ten years.

I'm grateful to the internet and my vagina is, too. I read about menstrual cups online and there are some great communities dedicated to them where women can ask questions, get advice, and share their experiences. The Diva Cup has changed my period from something I hate, dread, and fear into something I can handle and feel prepared for. It would have been scary to start using one on my own and I might not have. It's led to a better relationship with my vagina. And it really sucks that I can talk to hundreds of women online about it but only a few face to face.

—BECCA, 30, Illinois

In a study designed to investigate women's attitudes about these products, several gynecologists surveyed the patients in their clinic regarding their thoughts and opinions after reading a brochure for the product.[3] A total of sixty-nine patients completed the survey, of which 52 percent (thirty-six women) said that they would consider using the cup. The women found the cup appealing because it was better for the environment, required less-frequent changes, and eliminated the need to buy or carry supplies. In contrast, some women voiced concerns that the product would be messy, and others were uncomfortable about the fact that it required the use of one's hands to insert and remove. Nevertheless, it is important to keep in mind that these responses were from women who had never used the product. The reactions may have been quite different after the women had an opportunity to try menstrual cups for themselves. Have you given the product a try? Want to share your experiences? Let us and other readers know about your experience on our blog (www.readmylipsbook .tumblr.com) or Facebook page.

Menstrual sponges appear to be less popular than menstrual cups (at least they seem less widely available for sale on the Internet), but women have been using natural sponges for menstrual flow for ages. The key is that natural sponges are used—we're not talking about inserting kitchen-sink sponges inside your vagina, which would be unsanitary and potentially dangerous to the vagina and reproductive

---

PROMOTING PERIOD PRODUCTS

In 2010, Kotex won over a lot of fans—women and men alike—by making fun of typical feminine-product advertisements that depict periods as times for dancing, long walks on the beach, hearts, and rainbows (without actually ever showing a vulva diagram or even an actual tampon). Their slogan was, "Why are tampon ads so ridiculous?"

Well, they were not the first ones to ask this question. There are at least two analyses of tampon ads that were conducted to assess exactly what messages women receive from these types of advertisements. The first analysis from Dr. Debra Merskin[4] used feminine-hygiene advertisements from ten years' worth of teen magazines. She found that the majority of advertisements did not include a picture of a woman, and when they did, the woman was stationary (as opposed to engaging in an athletic or scientific activity). Most of the advertisements emphasized the comfort, ease, and bulkiness (or lack thereof) of the product. The advertisements addressed feelings of fear, secrecy, and freedom associated with menstruation/menstrual products.

In a later study, Drs. Simes and Berg[5] conducted an analysis of the content from two hundred women's magazines. They identified several themes throughout the articles, including silence and shame, embarrassment, ways to get caught (smelling like your period), ways to avoid getting caught (smelling fresh), and being constantly "dirty" while menstruating. Although the themes identified by both researchers were similar, one suggested that the ads were designed to dispel these negative perceptions, whereas the other suggested that these advertisements promoted women's negative feelings about their periods and their bodies. What do you think?

organs. Rather, sea sponges seem to be the sponge of choice when it comes to period flow. Of course, sponges are, well, spongy. Some women we've talked to have experienced period blood leakage when using menstrual sponges. Also, they need to be cleaned and preferably sterilized—such as in boiling water—after use, which can take time and is not always convenient (like if you're wanting to change your sponge while at work or school, or in a public restroom). Also, sea sponges commonly degrade over time and likely need to be replaced every few months if not more often.

Menstrual cups and sponges can be safe and "greener" alternatives to tampons and pads. However, because they are used over and over again in the vagina, they must be properly sanitized in between uses. Read the package insert that comes with your product for the most accurate and up-to-date directions regarding cleaning and sanitizing your cup or sponge. Some cups and sponges can be sanitized by boiling them in water for five to ten minutes and then left to air dry. Generally speaking, it is not recommended to use soapy products that may leave a residue on the cup or sponge, as the residue may irritate the vagina. Other cleaning agents that are generally NOT recommended for cup or sponge cleaning include tea tree oil, bleach, vinegar, peppermint castile soap, oil-based soaps, rubbing alcohol, hand sanitizer, dishwashing fluids, or soaps. Some of these may irritate the vagina, and some of them may compromise the integrity of silicone menstrual cups. Again: when in doubt, check your package insert or check with your healthcare provider for recommendations about cleaning agents or products that may be more likely to irritate the vagina so that you can avoid them.

THE SCENT OF A WOMAN

Recently, Always came out with a line of pads that included individually wrapped wipes for use between pads. As women, we have heard the message a million times before: your menstrual blood is dirty and needs to be covered up, and your vagina needs to be cleaned. It is an upsetting message given how natural menstrual blood is. Of course, we understand that people can get a little squeamish around blood, so we sympathize if menstrual blood brings about some of these feelings for the blood-phobic.

These handy little wipes do not only play sidekick to menstrual products. Advertisements encourage women to use an array of different products to get that "fresh feeling," including wipes, foams, and sprays. On the go? No problem! These products come in single-serving packages to take on the town with you in case you find yourself in a situation where you need your genitals to smell like fruit.

Okay, okay. We know a lot of people critique these products for making women feel bad about their genital smell. Rightfully so. We hate that women feel the need to conceal the natural scent of their genitals with the same scents that we would find in an air freshener. Still, if you are one of the women who use these products, we want you to know that we understand. With all these messages out there, it can be difficult not to feel self-conscious about one's genital odor.

VULVA IN A BOTTLE

Do you wish that your vulva smelled more like roses and less like a vulva? Perhaps this is because so many companies have pushed women to consider using flower-scented products to cover their natural feminine odor. However, what would you say if we told you there is a company that sells a product (of oil/lubricant consistency) that smells like a vulva? In fact, it's called Vulva. This is not a back-alley pervert product, either; it is marketed as classy and exotic, and selling for approximately 25 euros for two milliliters, it is also kind of pricey. Bottom line? The next time you are feeling self-conscious about your vulva smell, try to remember that some people would pay for just a sniff!

With so many of these products out there, do you ever wonder how many women are actually supporting this multi-million-dollar industry? Wonder no more! In Dr. Czerwinski's survey, she also asked about the use of other "feminine" products.[1] She found that older groups of women were actually more likely to use products than the younger women in the study. In the study, over 20 percent of women in the fifty-seven-and-up age group used feminine deodorant sprays and 40 percent used wet wipes. This is compared to only 8 percent of women in the under-forty-one age group who reported using feminine deodorant sprays and 26 percent who reported the use of wet wipes. In another study conducted several years later by our colleagues at the Indiana School of Medicine, Drs. Ott, Ofner, and Fortenberry found that these rates were actually much higher in the younger populations they studied.[6] They found that in a group of fourteen to eighteen-year-old women, 29 percent reported using feminine sprays and 27 percent reported using feminine wipes. Although they did not find that women who reported recent use were more likely to be diagnosed with an STI, they did find that the young women who reported an STI in their past were 1.7 times more likely to use feminine wipes. So, it remains unclear from this study whether product use was the cause or the effect.

That said, using these products may make it more difficult to diagnose a vaginal health problem. After all, some vaginal infections have a characteristic odor to them (such as a fishy odor) that can clue a doctor or nurse into what may be causing a woman's symptoms. If a woman covers up her vaginal odor with scented feminine-hygiene products, it may make it more difficult for her healthcare provider to realize that there's a problem or a possible infection that needs to be treated.

As such, whether you use feminine-hygiene products or not, consider steering clear of them before you go to the gynecologist. We know that they are tempting if you want to smell super special for your gynecologist, but remember that he/she is only concerned about your health and can miss something if you have recently used one of these products. If you use feminine-hygiene products at all, be sure to tell your gynecologist so that he/she can stay informed. The more he/

she knows about the things you do with your vagina and vulva, the better his/her help and advice will be.

We are not here to tell you what to do or make you feel bad about your choices. What we do want to do is give you all the information that you need to make an informed choice.

DOUCHE OR DON'T?

When Vanessa was in fourth grade, her babysitter broke the news to her: it was time to start douching. A little unusual? Although it does seem outside of the typical realm of babysitting duties, many women receive similar recommendations from the women in their lives. One study found that most women who douched learned about it from their mothers (45 percent), other female relatives (11.1 percent), friends (15.7 percent), or advertisements (11.7 percent).[7] Whether by commercial, magazine advertisements, family members, or (in Vanessa's case) babysitters, the fact is that many women learn from someone or somewhere that they are not naturally "clean" down there, and douching is recommended as the solution. It's too bad that these messages of vaginas being "dirty" or needing "cleaning" continue to be shared with women.

I wish women didn't feel so ashamed about the smell of their vaginas. So many of my friends tell me that they can't enjoy oral sex because they are always paranoid that they smell or taste badly or that they feel pressured to cum.

—JACQUIE, 28, Canada

Although people can douche in more ways than one, douches often look like a bag with a tube and nozzle attached. In order to douche, women typically fill the bag with water and insert the nozzle into their vaginas. Lift the bag up and—voila!—you have a steady douche. Some women use water, while others use marketed products, and a little over 5 percent of women use "home remedies."[7] Some of these self-made concoctions have included Lysol, hydrogen peroxide, tea tree oil, vinegar, yogurt, and Coca-Cola (yes, Coke)—none of which are recommended as they could cause vaginal irritation or other health problems.

Who Douches?

How many women do you think douche regularly? Take a guess. According to some of the latest national data (meaning that it includes people of various backgrounds, ages, geographic locations, etc.), just over 25 percent of women douche regularly,[8] down 10 percent from a decade earlier. These are averages and vary based on age and race, with about twice as many women in their twenties and thirties reporting douching than younger women. This may be because younger women are less interested in douching, have not started douching yet, or maybe even are not able to douche regularly if they are worried that a disapproving parent could catch them in the act. Most women who reported douching did it once or twice a month.[7]

Why Douche?

Every woman who douches probably has her reasons, but the most popular ones are to clean-up after periods or before/after sex, general hygiene, odor control, or just because it is what they think women do.[7]

On one hand, without any information, it seems to make sense. Without washing, the rest of our body can get pretty stinky. We even wash out our mouth and clean our ears. Why would our vagina be any different? Well, we'll tell you why. The vagina is a pretty magical place. It prepares itself for both sex and childbirth. In fact, one of its simplest tricks is its ability to keep itself clean (one of the few things that pussycats and pussy actually have in common).

Okay, so the vagina cleans itself. But the cleaner the better, right? Actually, no. The process of douching may remove normal vaginal flora (bacteria). If it seems that bacteria are something you normally want to get rid of, think again, as some bacteria are "good" in that they help to keep our bodies healthy. And anyway, your vagina is not a dirty kitchen counter. It is more like a wild flower; it is built to regulate itself and shouldn't be overwatered (and definitely not treated with Lysol or other kitchen disinfectants).

That isn't the only possible problem with douching. In addition to washing away good bacteria, douching can work as a not-so-fun little water slide, washing any potential issues (bad bacteria, STI) up past the cervix and into the uterus and the fallopian tubes. Numerous research studies have found that women who douche are more likely to be diagnosed with bacterial vaginosis, gonorrhea, chlamydia, pelvic inflammatory disease, cervical cancer, and HIV. They are also more likely to have higher infertility rates and ectopic pregnancies.[8] Does that mean that if you douche you are guaranteed to get an STI and have pregnancy difficulties? Of course not! It just means that your likelihood may be higher. So, when it comes to douching, our advice to most of you is "don't douche it!" Douching may help some women to feel more confident about their genital smell, taste, or health, or to

DOUCHING AS A FORM OF PREGNANCY PREVENTION

The condom breaks, he was supposed to pull out and missed the exit, you forgot the pill. We've heard them all, those stories that sent chills through the hearts of those who fear getting pregnant. Still, these things happen. If it happens to you, what do you do? Do you douche? In a certain way, it makes sense. You want that sperm out, and the douche will help get you clean quick, right? Wrong. The douche will squirt the sperm up, sending them on a joyride right toward their destination. So douching as a birth-control method is not recommended. Instead, try to reduce your pregnancy risk by using an effective method of contraception that works for you and condoms with sufficient lubrication. Emergency contraception (a.k.a. "the morning after pill") is a great back-up method should something not go as planned.

feel more generally "clean," and who are we to tell you what you should do or how you should feel? As with other health issues, if you have questions about douching and whether it is right for you, or how you can choose safer douches, this is a great topic to discuss with your OB/GYN or other healthcare provider. Remember: the more you tell your healthcare provider about your health practices, such as douching, the better he/she can handle your healthcare needs.

PRETTY IN PINK?

How many friends do you have who share the same skin color as you? No, no, we are not talking about race or ethnicity here. We mean the EXACT same color. Our guess is not many (if any). The same would probably be true if you were to compare the color of your inner labia.

Most inner labia are not just unique in terms of size and shape, they also vary in their color. Some are pink, some have purple hues, others are brown, and some are (or, with age, gradually turn) a bit gray. With few exceptions, no labia color is any better or healthier than others (one exception is that if you notice white patches of skin on your genitals, tell a healthcare provider, as this may signal a benign genital skin disorder that benefits from treatment; and if your labia or other vulva parts change in color, such as if they darken or develop moles, let a healthcare provider know so that he or she can examine them and make sure they are okay—more on this later in the chapter).

In our personal opinion, we feel that what is unique is beautiful. We once heard the colors of multicolored labia (it is sometimes a bit darker at the edges) described as being like a sunset. We love that image and are trying to reinforce comparisons between women's genitals and beautiful images in nature. As women, we are after all a part of nature, as well.

However, if in spite of reassurance from us or from your partner or healthcare provider you are still feeling concerned about the color of your inner labia, there is a new product that claims to restore the youthful look of your inner labia by making them pink. According to the product instructions, "A common concern amongst women about their labia minora (inside vaginal lips) and genital area, is the color loss and color change due to age, health, and many other factors. When the question is put to the female population about what color is most appealing to the eye, for their labia minora, the answer is 'Pink.' This is also the majority response amongst males for what is aesthetically appealing to the eye of their sexual partner."[9]

Even after disregarding the inaccuracy of this message (not all "young" women's inner labia are pink), we are still disturbed by the notion that only pink inner labia are attractive inner labia. That aside, although we may share our opinions in this book, we have a zero-judgment policy. Your vulva is your own, and you should be able to do with it whatever you would like. That being said, we do want you to be fully informed when doing it. We could think of no better way of doing that than giving the dye a try ourselves. Does it work? Does it burn? Does it result in a yeast infection? We wanted to give you a review you could trust.

We started the process by doing a spot test on our arms. We thought that this would be a good way to check for allergies and a fun way to tape the experience for your at-home enjoyment on our *Genitales* podcast. Long story short: it stung Debby's arm quite a bit and changed the color of her arm slightly. The discomfort, sting, and pain on her arm subsided after a few minutes, but it was enough for Debby to know that she didn't want this stuff anywhere near her labia.

Vanessa did not have much of an allergic reaction to it (or any noticeable results—the dye didn't seem to color her skin as much as it did Debby's skin, but then again, Debby has lighter skin than Vanessa). Because Vanessa had less of an adverse reaction during the spot test, it was decided that it was best for Vanessa to use it on its intended area: that's right, her labia. So, she did. The application process was quick and relatively easy given her comfort with and knowledge of her genitals. Unfortunately, the ease ended there. The process quickly turned from painless to what can best be described as sensations similar to that of an angry fire-ant colony attack on one's genitals. The sixty seconds required before it could be washed off could not come quickly enough. Thankfully, with water came quick relief. Once out of the shower and dry, Vanessa felt her labia were ready for inspection. She noted a discernable difference. Although the color we had chosen looked deep pink on the package, it managed to transform the labia a shade of red. If she didn't know any better, she would have guessed that her labia were just irritated (and we don't just mean mad because of the painful experience she underwent). It was definitely the dye—and it had definitely made a difference. That being said, hair-coloring rules likely apply here: you can go a shade darker, but this will not help you to go any lighter. So, the final recommendation: if you are

BLEACHING: AN ANAL-YSIS

Yes, we know this book is mostly about vulvas and vaginas and is not about the anus. Nevertheless, we thought this was an interesting topic and we figured, "Hey, the anus is the vulva's neighbor!"

So what color is your anal opening? If you answered, "I have no idea," then you are probably in good company. Many women (and men) have never given their anus a thorough anal-ysis before. For others, it can be a point of concern if they believe that it is too dark. Like the inner labia, there are dyes and lightening products available to address concerns about the color of one's anal opening. Some of these are applied in salons, and others can be applied at home on one's own. We've never tried these creams, but healthcare providers we know and trust generally do not recommend them (some suggest that certain lightening products may irritate the anal skin, which may, over time, lead to hyperpigmentation or darkening of the skin). Given the lack of evidence on the safety or side effects related to anal-bleaching products, we're not big fans. And anyway: your lover is probably just as clueless about the color of your anus as you are. Why not appreciate each other's parts instead of trying to change them?

not dissuaded by the Post-Traumatic Stress Disorder (PTSD) that your labia may endure following the coloring and are willing to risk the potential for pain or discomfort, then this product may "work" to dye labia a darker color. If you feel as though the color of your labia is fading, or if you just want to try a new color on for size, then this product may give you a color boost. If you are wanting to dye your labia a lighter color, this product is likely not for you. That's our honest review for you.

RECARPETING

"Does the carpet match the drapes?" As brunettes, we fortunately have avoided this question for most of our lives. Many redheaded and blonde ladies have not been so lucky. There are several famous examples of celebrities whose pubic hair color has been called into question based on the colors of the hair on their head (poor Lindsay).

The truth of the matter is that sometimes head hair and pubic hair match and other times they don't. For some women, it may not naturally match, and for others, it may not match because they dye their head hair, and others may go gray in one area before the other. Like the hair on our head, pubic hair comes in all different colors, all of which are beautiful. If you still feel self-conscious about your hair down there, we don't recommend using your typical hair dye in that sensitive area. It may be fine, but most hair dyes are not recommended for use on or near the genitals.

Purple Pubes?

That said, there is a new product line made specifically for dyeing pubic hair (see Resources). The owner claims to have come up with the idea while living in Europe. She said that she would notice salon customers lingering by the door, only to leave after the hairstylist approached them with a small brown bag of dye that they had mixed to match the hair on their head. The dye comes in "natural" colors, including blond, brown, and red. We particularly like their fun color line, which includes pink, purple, and bright green.

During a rebellious stage in high school, Vanessa used to dip into the bleach/blond hair dye and even played around with blue streaks. So the fun pubic hair dye colors brought back fond memories, and she volunteered to give it a try. We started with a spot test of the dye on Vanessa's leg. While this is often recommended to help detect if you are hypersensitive or allergic to a cosmetic product, we also did it for the benefit of the podcast. If you want to see the spot test and the results, check it out on our podcast at www.readmylipsthebook.tumblr.com. After twenty-four hours with no reaction from her leg-dyeing adventure, it was time for the real deal. The process was not terribly difficult, but it was time consuming. It involves two steps:

1. Bleach the hair blonde.
2. Dye the hair your color of choice (in this case, purple).

We learned a few lessons during the spot test that definitely helped during the actual test. First of all, it is important to *follow the directions*. This may seem obvious, but it is important and seemed worth repeating. Second, you want to coat every hair from root to tip. It is going to become obvious if you miss a spot. Finally, if you use the boosting tip to save time (covering the spot with cellophane wrap and blow-drying for five to ten minutes), it is important to make sure that your hairdryer has several heat and speed options. Put your hairdryer on a low speed and a medium heat setting, and be sure to keep the hairdryer moving. The improper use of the hairdryer (on high heat in one place) may have contributed to Vanessa experiencing a slight reaction following the bleaching stage. Other than that, Vanessa felt like a blonde down there for the first time in her life! It was a complete transformation.

The directions recommend using the dye immediately after the bleach. She considered following the "rules," but the first stage (being blond for once in her life) was so much fun that she waited a day before moving on to the dyeing-it-purple stage. The purple dyeing session went much more smoothly, as she'd learned from her previous mistake and was more careful with the hairdryer. In about ten minutes, she was in and out of the shower with a purple people eater all her own!

All in all, Vanessa felt that dyeing her pubes purple was a relatively easy process with surprisingly fun results. In addition to following the instructions (and considering our suggestions about hairdryer use above), we have a few additional tips/tricks:

- It is only recommended for use (as per the package insert) in a "safety zone." This zone includes your mons pubis. In other words, it is not for dyeing hair on the outer labia. This is important for safety reasons, as getting the dye closer to your inner labia or vaginal opening could cause significant irritation. Thus, it is perhaps best used by those who want to stencil in a design or change the color of the hair on the mons—or who are into two-toned hair (dyed hair in the safety zone and natural color hair elsewhere).
- If you are not careful, it will dye your skin along with your hair. Don't panic, the dye should wash off of your skin in a day or less. This may be helpful to know in case you are introducing someone new to the color or to your vulva for the first time. If that is the case, you may want to dye your hair at least twenty-four hours in advance in preparation/anticipation.
- If you are deciding between the blond and another color, we recommend the color! As mentioned, the process of coloring your pubic hair involves dyeing it blond first anyway. We think that getting the color is like a little freebie: two colors (blond plus a fun color, such as purple, green, pink) for the price of one.

Women's pubic hair comes in all shapes, sizes, lengths, textures, and colors. Try not to stress if you think that your pubic hair is unusual. However, if you like the idea of unusual pubic hair, there are now plenty of color options for you to try—a definite option when lingerie gets old and you are feeling bold!

I wish more women knew that porn is airbrushed, and whatever size or color or shape their genitals are is just lovely. We (men especially, I think) have been conditioned to think that women's genitals should be perfectly coiffed (or hairless), that the labia should be even and not too long, and that the clitoris should be straight. That's ridiculous.

—TAYLOR, 25, Illinois

DOES ONE SIZE FIT ALL?

Vanessa used to have a friend who would always joke begrudgingly that "it was just her luck that her vagina was the only small part of her body." That statement always struck Vanessa as a little funny because she had always been under the impression that, like most other parts of the body, women were supposed to believe that "less is more" when it comes to their vaginal circumference. Isn't it the common cultural idea for women to have a vagina that's "tight" (a.k.a. small)?

Fortunately, no. Women and their vaginas come in all shapes and sizes—and men and women who partner with women have a range of likes and preferences, too. Many women have probably never checked out their vaginal size in any detail. Those who have considered their vaginal size may have done so in relation to a partner. For instance, depending on your "fit" with your partner, you may wish that your vagina had a slightly wider circumference for more comfortable sex if your partner is quite large or a narrower circumference if your partner is on the slimmer side. (Or you may have wished that your male partner's penis was a little smaller or bigger to enhance your genital fit or sensation during sex.)

We understand thinking/feeling this way at times. We also understand that where there is a market, there will be a product to fill it (literally, in this case). Although we understand the reasons for the products, we do not have to agree with the marketing tactics used to promote some of them. For instance, there are vaginal creams that claim to make you feel "like a virgin" again. Who would want that? We can't imagine that many women would want to undergo the fear and pain that they may have experienced when "losing" their virginity the first time. We also worry that such products may make some women feel badly about their vagina and its size. Disapprove. Then again, we are well aware that many women struggle with issues related to how they feel about their vaginal size or sensation, perhaps especially after having children. We get it. And we definitely believe that healthcare providers should be more attentive to women's questions about their vaginas, including how vaginas and vulvas may change due to pregnancy or childbirth. Far too many women feel brushed aside by their doctors who tell them things like, "Once you have a baby, nothing is ever the same again—including your vagina." Who benefits from a line like that?

Marketing messages aside (they don't all share the same message), what do we think of vaginal-tightening products? Well, Vanessa has been pretty brave and has experimented quite a bit with the products out there, but we were extra wary about this one. Most of the products contain potassium alum. Have you ever used or seen natural rock deodorant from the health-food store? Well, that's a great example of potassium alum—not something that we were excited to insert in our vaginas. That being said, we did peruse the reviews for some time before we came to that decision. If all the reviews are real, they ranged from "it increased my and my partner's sexual pleasure" to "it did nothing" to "it dried me out" to "it gave me a yeast infection." Sure it may work—but it sounds risky.

Also, we had heard from some of our colleagues who are doctors and others who sell sex toys and other sexual-enhancement products that many of the vaginal-tightening creams work by inflaming the vagina. That didn't sound at all fun to us. Rather than risking irritation or inflammation to our vaginas or yours, why not opt for Kegel exercises, which can help to tone the pelvic-floor muscles? For decades, these exercises have helped many women with genital sensation. That said, we realized that some women feel as though Kegels only do so much for them. In these cases, women should ask their healthcare providers, or a physical therapist who has training in genital-health issues and the pelvic-floor muscles, what else may be done to improve their perceptions of their genital size or genital sensation.

At the Other End of the Spectrum

We started off this section by pointing out that women vary in how they feel about their vaginal size and circumference. Of course, this doesn't mean that all women wish that they were smaller. We want to make sure that we don't leave out our ladies who long for a larger circumference or a more comfortable genital fit with a male partner.

If you are hoping to increase your vaginal circumference to ease intercourse with a more endowed male partner, we recommend the following:

1. Don't be too hard on yourself. Take it easy and relax—the more nervous you are, the tighter and less lubricated you may be.
2. Spend at least ten minutes in foreplay, which can help your vagina to tent and create more space.
3. Use lots and lots and lots of lubrication. It can make vaginal penetration more comfortable and easier.
4. Try to ease into it. Have a partner ease in one finger at a time and move it around until you find an arousing angle. Once you are comfortable, ease in another finger and repeat. If you have a few sex toys that are narrower in girth, it may help to get started with those.

These little tricks should have you eased into a more pleasurable sexual experience in no time. If you still find vaginal penetration difficult or even impossible, we recommend that you check in with a healthcare provider. Occasionally, various medical or anatomical issues can make penetration more difficult. Some of these conditions can be easily treated to make penetration a more comfortable possibility. Finally, if you feel as though your vagina is too small for comfortable penetration with tampons, fingers, sex toys, or a male partner's penis—don't despair. Dilator use (described in detail in chapter 4) may be of benefit to you.

A Different Type of Hole

Whoever said that women's genitals only have three holes clearly did not get her vulva pierced. This section would not be complete without a brief section on genital piercing. Although slightly more common for males, there are certainly many women who have a pierced poonanny. The safety of these piercings varies, and there is little regulation over the procedures. As you can imagine, then, people who choose to have their genitals pierced are taking a risk and would be well advised to talk with their healthcare providers and ask questions before doing so.

What we can tell you about are some of the most popular piercing styles.[10] Piercings through the outer labia can take longer to heal (two to four months) than clitoral or inner-labia piercings (two to six weeks). The most common piercings are through the clitoral hood, the body of the clitoris, or the inner or outer labia. Oftentimes, women will opt for several piercings. As you can imagine, the clitoral piercings are said to increase sexual sensation. In fact, it is likely not just sexual sensation, but also sensation when at the office, grocery store, and everywhere in between. Do you decorate down there? Do you love it? Hate it? Does it give you pleasure? An infection? Tell us about it on our web site or Facebook page.

If you or your partner has a genital piercing, you may find it easier to start sex slowly. If your piercing can be removed and put back in, you may want to remove your piercing(s) before having intercourse or oral sex (yes, there have been cases in which piercings have chipped teeth or been accidentally swallowed). Condom use can be challenging, too, as piercings may tear the condoms. As such, make sure to get screened for STIs before having sex together, just in case the male or female condom breaks or in case you choose to forgo condoms altogether.

PRODUCTS?

Love it or hate it, the vulva has been a source of revenue for many people—and we're not talking about prostitution here. Some products are simply modern translations of products that have been around for thousands of years; others probably address realistic wants/needs/desires of women, and other companies may create a need for a product or a service that no one ever cared about before its existence (and marketing). Regardless of how you feel about the products, we are hoping this chapter armed you with the information you need to make a choice about what (if any) product is right for you.

TEST YOUR VQ

1. When do doctors recommend that an average woman should douche?
   a. as frequently as she can—the cleaner the better!
   b. once a month after she finishes her period
   c. after sex as a form of birth control
   d. never ever

2. Which of the following statements is true about tampons?
   a. They may take your virginity.
   b. Some expand lengthwise while others expand widthwise.
   c. There is a likelihood that you will get TSS if left in for too long.
   d. If you push your tampon too hard, it can get lost inside of your body.

3. Inner labia that are not pink
   a. are considered unattractive
   b. only occur after menopause
   c. indictate a health issue
   d. are very common

Answers

1. d
2. b
3. d

· 6 ·

The Hair Down There

$\mathcal{T}$hink back to when you first remember becoming aware of the fact that girls, as they develop into young women, develop hair on their genitals (let alone their underarms and perhaps thicker hair on their legs). You may have seen a drawing that illustrated the kinds of body changes you could expect to see on girls and boys. Maybe you used to shower or bathe with your mother and noticed that her genitals looked different than yours, particularly in regard to the hair on hers or how she used a razor on her genitals whereas you, as a child without pubic hair, didn't do this as part of bathing. Or maybe no one told you or showed you anything about puberty as it pertains to pubic hair. Like many girls on the verge of womanhood, perhaps the first time you knew anything about pubic hair was when it first began to appear on your own genitals. Alternatively, the first time pubic hair appeared on your radar screen may have been when, on *Sex and the City*, Charlotte got a Brazilian wax, Samantha freaked out over a gray pube, or the girls suggested that Miranda—married and having infrequent sex with her husband, Steve—trim things up down there.

Men: Back off the hair. Seriously. I am very positive about my body, and I can only imagine how these jerks affect women who are less positive or unsure. This belongs to me!

—RACHEL, 32, New Mexico

Women recall varied experiences relating to first becoming aware of pubic hair. Some women remember feeling horrified or embarrassed about pubic hair as it began sprouting on their genitals. At least one woman we know used to sneak her mother's razor in order to get rid of the hair that she didn't realize was a natural part of puberty and thus didn't fully understand. Other women remember feeling proud and happy about their pubertal changes, including their genital changes, feeling as though they were going through a momentous and special change that would soon enough turn them into grown women.

One mom we know talked to us about her daughter's process of pubertal change. As a mom who is knowledgeable about sex and comfortable talking about it, she raised her daughter in a home environment that fostered developmentally appropriate conversations about gender, sexuality, and pubertal changes. When her daughter began developing pubic hair, she would count her new pubic hairs. Not only that, but much to her mother's surprise, she would report new hair growth—with great joy and pride—to her mother, who would congratulate her on her development. "I have six hairs now!" she would say over breakfast, as if telling her mom about receiving a good grade on an exam. If only all girls were raised in such open, supportive homes! And if only all women could continue to feel proud about their bodies rather than feeling as though they have to tweak them to meet the (real or imagined) approval of their doctors, partners, or a standard set by magazines.

I think that it is important to talk about our vulvas, vaginas, clitori, labias, and pubic hair out loud and in public. Men have been talking about their respective genitals since men could speak, and they do so in the television, on the radio, on the cross-town bus, at the bar, in mixed company, at family reunions, and so on. So I think it is time we took some of the mystery and silence out of female genitalia. Women's bodies aren't dirty and shameful and it is time that the world realizes it.

—SAMANTHA, 28, Michigan

In this chapter, we'll describe the many things that women have done to their pubic hair throughout different historical time periods and in different cultures, including what we know from Greek vase painting, Egyptian art, and nudes of the Northern Italian Renaissance (who had hair, who didn't, and why). You'll learn about a research study we conducted that involved asking more than twenty-five hundred women about their pubic hair. In this study, we asked women what they do with their pubic hair (Shave it? Wax it? Leave it alone?) and how much they remove (if any), and we also looked at patterns to understand how women's pubic hairstyles relate to their sex lives and how they feel about their genitals. The data were surprising to us, and we hope they will be of interest to you, too. We'll also take a look at merkins of yesteryear in addition to modern-day salon offerings such as vajazzling, vajacials, and vatooing. Although pubic hair isn't a new invention, some of the things people do down there are. Consider this the ultimate guide to your pubes.

OUR HERSTORY IN HAIR

Pubic hair doesn't have as much of a recorded herstory as, say, how women's bodies or hairstyles (on their head) have evolved over time. After all, bodies and hairstyles are publicly viewable. For centuries, when women were drawn, painted, turned into sculptures or—in more recent times—photographed or filmed, they were mostly done so wearing clothes. Consequently, while their bodies and hairstyles were evident, their pubic hair was typically not visible. As such, it's not entirely clear how women's pubic hairstyles have changed over time. We only have a handful of sources, such as literature and paintings, that give us any hint at all about what our female ancestors did to their pubic hair.

WHAT'S HAIR FOR, ANYWAY?

As humans didn't invent pubic hair—it's been there all along as far as we can tell—it's a little unclear to scientists why exactly we have pubic hair. Some think that it may help to trap pheromones, which may help us to unconsciously connect with people we're attracted to. Others suggest that pubic hair helps to create a sort of "padding" during intercourse to reduce friction between two people's bodies. It may also help to keep our reproductive parts somewhat warmer.

Women were shown with triangular areas of pubic hair in ancient Egyptian art, and Greek literature suggests that women engaged in at least some form of pubic hair grooming, such as plucking hairs or singeing them with a lamp.[1] Also, there is some suggestion that the presence of pubic hair on women's bodies was considered sexually attractive. The reasons why the women depicted in Italian Renaissance art appear with no pubic hair and the women depicted in art from Northern Italy, and in Gothic art, appear to have some pubic hair is not clear.[2] Were there differences in women's pubic hairstyles in these places and times? Or did the (often male) artists paint women's genitals as they *imagined* them—regardless of what women often looked like nude? We don't know. The German Renaissance artist Lucas Cranach the Elder often depicted women's genitals in rather vague ways. Sometimes they were covered with leaves and/or branches, as in *Adam and Eve* (1528) and *The Close of the Silver Age* (approximately 1527–1535). In other paintings, such as *Venus Standing in a Landscape* (1529) and *Venus and Amor* (1534), the mons is visible but lacks detail—there are no pubic hairs to speak of, but then again, there is also no hint of labia (e.g., a "slit" or "camel toe").

It's not always clear to what extent the artists had experience with women as nude models or if they simply imagined what women looked like naked. Also, artists who did have nude female models available to them may have been more likely to have prostitutes or courtesans model for them, and these women's pubic hairstyles may have differed from other women in their towns. Women with many sex partners, such as prostitutes and courtesans, would have been at greater risk for pubic lice (as they are even today), and removing one's pubic hair is one way to protect oneself from pubic-lice transmission, a tactic that some suggest was widely practiced by sex workers of the time for this reason.[3, 4] After all, if a person (male or female) doesn't have pubic hair, then even if they're exposed to pubic lice (crabs), there are no hairs for the lice to cling to.

In the late nineteenth century, Goya's painting *The Naked Maja* featured a nude woman with sparse pubic hair reclining on a lounge chair. But it was Gustave Courbet's *L'Origine du Monde* (1866; translated as *The Origin of the World*) that eventually—at least when it was publicly exhibited—caused a bit of a stir by prominently featuring a woman's genitals in detail, with a full mound of pubic hair and the outer labia (labia majora). (Note: this painting was originally created for a benefactor's private collection and passed through several private collections before becoming a part of various museum collections and being seen by the masses.) This painting didn't just depict the origin of babies' worlds, as per conception and vaginal birth; it also—at least in hindsight—hinted at a world in which women's genitals would (eventually) begin to be more openly displayed. Or, at least, we like to think of it this way. The image has been reprinted in several books and has continued to be a source of controversy, at times challenging community standards of decency.

THE NOT-SO-PERFECT PUBIC STORM

As fascinating as the herstory of pubic hair from days gone by can be, many people are interested in the state of pubic hair in more contemporary times—and for good reason, as it's an interesting story! Though the media often focus on the dawn of the Brazilian in the 1990s in New York City, or on the frequent images of young,

V-CRAFT: MAKE YOUR OWN MERKIN

If it's not already abundantly clear, we are big fans of the vulva and of women's rights to make choices about their own bodies and sexualities. In short, we think you should style, keep, or remove your pubic hair in whatever way makes you happy. If you want to grow a long, thick, natural mane (the better to run your fingers sensually through), we've got your back. We'll also high-five you if you prefer to keep your pubic hair trimmed or shaved into shapes, or if you remove every last hair on your mons, labia, inner thighs, and around your anal area. If you're down with your down there, we think that's great.

Whether you have hair and think it would be fun to have even more or you're bare and would occasionally like to masquerade around with some, here's how you can make your own merkin (a.k.a. a pubic wig). Many people think that prostitutes who would go bare to treat or prevent pubic lice created merkins. However, now they are used mainly for fun, or in Hollywood movies to mask actresses' genitals or for period pieces in which the female characters would have had full, natural pubic hair rather than neat landing strips or some other design.

Before proceeding with this craft, you may want to watch Amanda Palmer's music video "Map of Tasmania" for inspiration (it's available on YouTube the last time we checked; "map of Tasmania" is apparently Australian slang for a woman's pubic area).

What You'll Need

- A cotton thong or G-string, the thinner and stringier the sides, the better. Your merkin will look more natural if the thong or G-string matches the color of the skin on your hips/stomach.
- A wig—often available at arts-and-crafts shops or costume shops. Choose whatever color (Brown? Black? Red? Purple?) or texture

often panty-less female celebrities being photographed up their skirts as they exit cars, there is much more to the story of vulvas and pubic hair than these elements. Join us as we take a brief tour through the past few decades of pubes.

(Short and curly? Straight and smooth?) you prefer. Wigs can work better than free-standing hair or weaves because the hair is already sewn into some type of fabric or cap.

- glue
- scissors
- marker

What to Do

1. Hold the triangular pubic area of your thong/G-string up to the back fabric-side of your wig.
2. Trace the triangular part of the underwear onto the fabric side of the wig.
3. Cut the wig along the lines you've traced.
4. Place glue on the fabric side of the wig, then press it onto the triangular part of your thong or G-string underwear on the part facing out.

If you're good at sewing, you might find that sewing the triangular piece of the wig to your G-string provides a more secure fit than gluing it.

You can wear your merkin at home alone for fun. Alternatively, you can wear it for a partner and encourage him or her to rub their fingers through your new set of hair. A homemade merkin also serves as quite the conversation piece when worn as part of a costume (wear tights underneath your merkin if you'd like to cover more skin or are worried it might slip to the side, thus revealing your genitals).

Note, too, that you can switch the wig out for any kind of materials that you prefer: cotton balls, Legos, yarn, hair curlers, or fake flowers or leaves (frequently sold at craft stores) are all options. Use your imagination!

NOTABLE MOMENTS IN PUBIC HAIR

1972: Dr. Benjamin Nair invents a depilatory cream, now known as "Nair," that is marketed for hair removal.

1979: Artist Judy Chicago first exhibits her installation *The Dinner Party*, featuring thirty-nine place settings and china plates (many of the latter featuring vulvas) for historical and mythical women. Being somewhat abstract, it's unclear whether most of the vulvas have pubic hair.[5]

1982: Full, natural pubic hair is on display in the naked college-coed shower scene made famous in *Porky's*.

1985: Designer Rudi Gernreich—already known for inventing the monokini—unveiled the pubikini, a bathing suit for women that featured a small V-shaped strip to show off women's pubic hair.

1989: The Cunt Coloring Book is published, giving artistic license for women (and men) to create their Dream Vulvas—hairstyles included.

1992: In her role in *Basic Instinct*, Sharon Stone reveals her vulva in a famous (but brief) leg-crossing scene, leading to a great deal of curiosity about her hairstyle. Reports circulated suggesting that she did not realize her vulva would be shown in the movie, making this an early instance of non-consensual female upskirt shots in Hollywood.

1996: The Vagina Monologues, written by and starring Eve Ensler, debuts at HERE Arts Center in New York. One monologue is titled "Hair."[6]

1998: Betty Dodson releases *Viva La Vulva*, a video that highlights interviews with women about their genitals and, as part of the genital portraits, features pubic hair grooming and styling.[7]

The Vagina Monologues author Eve Ensler launches V-Day, a campaign to end violence against women and girls that involves women on college campuses and cities around the world mounting performances of *The Vagina Monologues* as fundraising events. Consequently, thousands of women begin talking more openly about vaginas and selling products, such as T-shirts with the word "vagina" on them and chocolate-vulva lollipops. There is some controversy over how many of the "vaginas" mentioned in the play are actually vulvas, and there is much continued dialogue about hair.

2000: The Brazilian wax—already somewhat trendy thanks to quotes surfacing from actress Gwyneth Paltrow about how waxing changed her life—is featured on *Sex and the City*.

2003: Photographer Mario Testino shoots model Carmen Kass, mostly naked and with her underwear pulled down to reveal her pubic hair shaved into the letter G (for Gucci). Some called for the ad image—dubbed "Pubic Enemy"—to be banned.

2004: The V Book: A Doctor's Guide to Complete Vulvovaginal Health[8] is published along with information about pubic hair removal methods.

2006: Brandon Davis uses the word "firecrotch" to describe Lindsay Lohan in an online video. The video gets picked up and the term is, sadly, used persistently by gossip blogger Perez Hilton in posts about Lohan.

2005: In a *New York Times* article titled "The Revised Birthday Suit," writer Natasha Singer speaks to women opting for a more permanent "baldness" down there, via laser hair-reduction treatments. There are also mentions of men going bare, women dyeing their pubic hair pink, and a woman with a lightning bolt pattern to her pubes.

2006: In separate incidents, the bare vulvas of Paris Hilton, Lindsay Lohan, and Britney Spears are photographed and appear on Hollywood gossip blogs.

Just speaking the words vagina, pussy, genitals, clitoris without hesitation is a huge leap! I think we as women give permission to other women to feel comfortable, maybe that seems obvious but I rarely spoke the words even to my girls. I care if a man might feel turned off and not want to have oral sex because he thinks I'm not like some picture at times, but deep down I think most men are not that picky. I think fear can crush some sweet girls out there. I guess that we as women need to shift from thinking about our bodies only for sex and remember health and happiness comes first . . . sex follows.

—ELLEN, 53, New Jersey

In *The Break Up*, Brooke (played by Jennifer Aniston) gets a Brazilian wax and then—to induce jealousy or to get revenge—
walks around naked in the apartment she's sharing with the
boyfriend she's recently split from, played by Vince Vaughn.

Two physicians in the UK, Dr. Armstrong and Dr. Wilson,
publish a letter in the journal *Sexually Transmitted Infections*
titled "Did the Brazilian Kill the Pubic Louse?" The doctors
note that although rates of chlamydia and gonorrhea increased
in their practice from 1997 to 2003, the rates of pubic lice
(crabs) decreased, particularly around 2000 (for women) and
2003 (for men), coinciding with the popularity of Brazilian
waxing.[9]

2007: Body Drama by Nancy Redd is published as a book for
younger women. It is body-affirming, featuring many images of
diverse bodies—including vulvas. In fact, there are twenty-four
images of vulvas laid side by side with varied pubic hairstyles
including fancy fluffs, groomed lady gardens, and beautiful
bare-naked lady parts. (Well, we came up with these terms; but
you get the picture—the women in her photos do all sorts of
fun things with their hair.)

Hank Moody sings the praises of women's natural pubic hair (and
natural labia) on the popular show, *Californication*.

Debby takes her Wondrous Vulva Puppet on *The Tyra Banks Show*
to teach women about their genital parts in an episode called
"What's Up Down There?" The clip goes viral to millions of
viewers on YouTube, in part because of it being posted on
PerezHilton.com and aired on *Talk Soup* and *Best Week Ever*.
And yes, pubic hairstyles get a nod.

The movie *Knocked Up* features a famous birth scene in which
the main character, played by Katherine Heigl, gives birth and
her vulva is completely bare. The blogosphere chatters away
about the bald "stunt vulva."

Reality show actor Spencer Pratt allegedly writes a negative post
about actress Lauren Conrad (LC), describing her as having

"beef curtains." Perez Hilton runs with this term and frequently calls LC by that name afterward.

Finnish performance artist Mimosa Pale launches her "Mobile Female Monument," which she describes as "an interactive performance sculpture on wheels." It's also known as a large vulva sculpture operating as a bicycle taxi. Her "bicycle bits," as we like to think of them, were on exhibit at the Tennispalatsi Art Museum in Helsinki, where they were taken for a walk around town every other day. Individuals could enter the sculpture, and there was reportedly enough room for an adult to lie down in it. (See MimosaPale.com for photos.)[10]

2008: Rachel Liebert founds the International Vulva Knitting Circle (IVKC), a "grass-roots activist collective in support of the New View Campaign's WTF-ing against the emerging industry of female genital cosmetic surgeries." In its first year, the IVKC had almost 150 diverse knit vulvas from five countries.

Comedian and author Amy Sedaris appears on Chelsea Handler's show, *Chelsea Lately*, and teaches Chelsea about "vaginal cleansing" using a model that she says was made by Todd Oldham. Though there are some wavy lines on the outside of what she calls the "outer folds" (the outer labia, we presume), it's unclear if these are meant to be pubic hairs or not.

2009: Actress Kate Winslet tells *Allure* about wearing a merkin for her role in *The Reader*. "I had to grow the hair down there," she said. "But because of years of waxing . . . it doesn't come back quite the way it used to. They even made me a merkin—a wig—because they were so concerned that I might not be able to grow enough."

The New View Campaign holds an event titled "Vulvagraphics: An Intervention in Honor of Female Genital Diversity" at The Change You Want to See Gallery in Brooklyn, New York. The event features vulva-related art including knit vulvas from the IVKC.

The UK newspaper *The Guardian* publishes an article featuring the work of "The Muffia"—two female performance artists, Sinead King and Katie O'Brien, who lift their dresses and expose merkin-covered underwear while communicating messages to passersby. These messages raise questions about women's issues, such as female genital cosmetic surgery, eating disorders, and more.

2010: The Hairy Underwear Collection is founded on January 4, 2010, by Finnish duo the Nutty Tarts (tarahtaneet.net) and features underwear that are given the appearance of having pubic hair on the crotch.

On *Lopez Tonight*, actress Jennifer Love Hewitt talks about getting vajazzled. "After a breakup, a friend of mine Swarovski crystalled my, um, precious lady," Hewitt told Lopez. "It shined like a disco ball."

VATOOING

We would rather this be called a "vulvoo," rather than a "vatoo"—as it's not actually a temporary tattoo for the vagina but for the vulva. And in all fairness, it's also been called a "vatu" and a "twatoo" in the blogosphere. Essentially, the vatoo is an airbrushed image toward the top of, or just above, a woman's waxed-bare mons, and it was pioneered by the Completely Bare salon in Manhattan.

Although a fun and kind of quirky idea, one video we watched about vatoos had the aesthetician warning not to mess it up during sex. This doesn't bode well for sex positions such as the coital alignment technique, a variation on missionary that involves a woman and her partner lining their bodies up quite closely and grinding, rather than thrusting in and out. Coital alignment technique has been shown to help make it easier for women to experience orgasm during intercourse. Given the choice between a no-holds-barred sex act and a not-smudged vatoo, which would you take?

In a *New York Times* profile of the J Sisters (who reportedly started the Brazilian-wax trend), writer Stephanie Clifford attributes the decline of the Brazilian to the 2008 recession.

Vanessa and Debby take to the Las Vegas Strip with Vanessa dressed up as a giant vulva, a costume she made herself. This occurs the evening before the New View Campaign's conference at the University of Nevada Las Vegas called *Framing the Vulva: Genital Cosmetic Surgery and Genital Diversity* (newview campaign.org).[11]

In her book *Chelsea Chelsea Bang Bang*, Chelsea Handler writes about learning about her genitals—what she calls her "coslopus" and likens to a pincushion—while growing up. When she learned that she would one day grow pubic hair on her coslopus, she says that she experienced mixed feelings about this and would frequently wonder, in a way that only Chelsea can do, "Pubic hair or pincushion by itself?"

2011: Groupon airs a Super Bowl commercial featuring model Elizabeth Hurley in which she begins by talking about the perils of deforestation impacting the Brazilian rainforest—that is, before she says, "but not all deforestation is bad." The example she uses is that "since 100 of us bought at Groupon .com, we're all saving 50 percent on a Brazilian wax at Completely Bare in New York City."

WHAT DO WOMEN DO DOWN THERE, ANYWAY?

Not long ago, our research team at Indiana University conducted a study about women's pubic hair-removal patterns. Like many people, we were curious about what women were doing with their pubic hair. We had read many magazine articles that claimed that nearly all young women were going bare. We even came across articles that said going bare was increasingly common among women from their mid-twenties to their forties and fifties. But this didn't make much sense to us.[12]

WHAT'S YOUR STYLE?

"I prefer to have a 'tuft' of pubic hair on my mons pubis, and keep my labia majora as hairless as possible. I like how this looks, and it decreases my frequency of yeast infections. My partner also likes this style because it is easier for him to perform oral sex on me."—Alana, 22, Indiana

"Bald, smooth, shaved top to bottom. It is what I have always liked."—Zoe, 36, Canada

"Have shaved completely in the past because of partner's preference. Currently shave vulva and keep mons hair short."—Abby, 28, Texas

"I trim, but not shave. I don't think this is influenced by anyone's preference besides my own."—Rachel, 25, Colorado

"I prefer to have a nicely manicured triangle at the top and hair-free labia. It's due to my preferences. I love to touch the bare labia."—Gina, 36, Washington

"I've often trimmed it but also leave it ungroomed often. One lover shaved my pubic hair. I really liked how it felt, but it was inconvenient to maintain. Also, if I shaved my pubic hair now, I'd be self-conscious in the locker room. Most of my lovers haven't expressed a preference."—Casey, 43, Indiana

"Busy, with the 'hedges'—hair that extends past my panty line, removed."—Jill, 36, New York

"My pubic hair is waxed into a 'California' strip. My labia majora and mons pubis both have hair on them (that I keep trimmed), but the bikini line, plus a bit extra is waxed off. My partner doesn't care one way or another how I have my pubic hair. I just like feeling clean and able to wear a bathing suit without being embarrassed by hair sticking out everywhere."—Mary, 31, Texas

"Trimmed (sometimes VERY short and other times just a bit). I have no pain tolerance and am irrationally afraid of taking a razor to that area (no clue why but I am)! However, going wild and free is a little itchy so I give it a haircut. I remember making a pact with a friend in high school to never do anything to our vulvas for a partner . . . only for us based on what we want! While this, in hindsight, is a little extreme, when I was rocking full bush and my partner didn't love it . . . I told him OH WELL, I don't expect it of you and I'm kind of loving it (until I didn't anymore)!"—Hilary, 22, Massachusetts

"I leave my pubic hair completely alone. Sometimes for fun I will trim—and one time I tried shaving it all—but generally I just leave it. I do however have very little hair and when it's completely grown out it still doesn't show outside my bikini bottoms. As for my friends . . . definitely everyone grooms, if not waxing or laser. My friends and I talk about it sometimes but I am in no way interested in grooming my pubic hair constantly. My partner prefers when I'm completely grown out."—Jessica, 28, Canada

"Prefer it all shaved/waxed. I'm not fond of body hair on me or on anyone else."—Kali, 22, India

"I prefer it slightly waxed so it doesn't show in a bathing suit. I disagree with Brazilians. I wish grown women didn't want to look like 10 year old girls."—Jane, 48, New York

"I don't care much how it looks. I enjoy cutting hair so it's fun to mess with. I also tried trimming it to get my girlfriend to want to go down on me more. Didn't work, however."—Anne, 26, Idaho

"When I was with my first partner I hadn't had sex before so I didn't know of his expectations. I left my genital hair natural and he was very surprised when he first saw it, he said something along the lines of 'it's hairier than mine' (which wasn't even true) and I think he expected that I'd naturally have very little hair there or none at all. For this reason I shaved it off while I was with him. When I broke up with him I decided that it was a stupid expectation and that I actually preferred to have some hair there as shaving is uncomfortable, so now I just trim and shave around it but leave most of the hair where it naturally should be!"—Liz, 22, UK

"Completely shaved, obviously affected by society, but I personally like the feel of it bare and shave even when I am not planning on having anyone see it. My partner definitely likes it shaved, but if he didn't I wouldn't grow it because hair feels scratchy and uncomfortable to me down there."—Cynthia, 18, Connecticut

"There is no peer pressure for a woman of my age to be waxed or shaven but since I was in my twenties I have trimmed my pubic hair and had electrolysis on the bikini line or waxing. These days I only trim as I wear skimpy clothing less. I do pluck the odd hair from the groin area."—Brenda, 55, Australia

In part, this didn't hold up because Debby often teaches human sexuality classes to college students at Indiana University, and they had more diverse stories to tell. When the topic of pubic hair removal would come up in class or in students' papers, she learned that these young women described a wide range of things they did with their pubic hair. Some kept it natural. Others trimmed. And still others shaved, waxed, or used more permanent methods (such as laser hair reduction). We had also talked about pubic hairstyles with friends and found that they did different things with their hair, too. And being in a locker room, one can see a range of styles.

We found that there was very little scientific data on the subject and decided to conduct our own study of women's pubic-hair removal patterns as part of a larger study we were conducting related to women's sexuality. We published the results of our study in the *Journal of Sexual Medicine* in 2010 and are happy to share them with you here as well.

In total, we asked 2,451 women ages eighteen to sixty-eight, to tell us whether, how, and how often they had removed their pubic hair over the previous month.[12] We asked about shaving, waxing, laser hair reduction, and electrolysis. We also asked how much hair they removed (some or all of it). Then we categorized women into groups based on what their pubic hair had been like over the previous month—did they remove all of it so often that they were likely bare most or all of the time? If so, we called them "typically hair-free." If they removed all of their hair only a few times, we described them as engaging in "some total removal." Women who removed some, but never all, of their pubic hair were grouped as "some removal, not total." Everyone else fell into the category of not having used any of the removal methods we asked about.

Now, this wasn't a perfect study. We didn't, for example, ask about depilatory creams, which some women may use on their genitals. But it was the largest study ever conducted on women's pubic-hair removal patterns and covered a lot of different age groups, so we're quite proud of it, even if it wasn't perfect.

HAIR, BARE, AND EVERYWHERE: WHAT WE LEARNED

What we found is that going bare isn't nearly as common as many media reports suggest. Even among the youngest age group in our study (women ages eighteen to twenty-four), only 20.6 percent of women were typically bare. Another third (38.0 percent) removed all of their pubic hair some of the time, which means that some of the time they had pubic hair. We can't help but wonder if these women remove their pubic hair only if they expect to have sex or when they have a GYN exam, as we know from other research we've conducted that women commonly groom their pubic hair before they see their doctor. Nearly one-third of college-aged women (29.1 percent) reported removing some, but never all, of their pubic hair over the previous month. The rest (12.4 percent) didn't remove any of it that we know of.[12]

Women in older age groups were even less likely to remove all of their pubic hair. Among women ages twenty-five to twenty-nine:

- 12.4 percent were typically hair-free (went bare much of the time)
- 32.2 percent were sometimes hair-free
- 39.4 percent removed some of their hair, such as through waxing or shaving, but never all of it
- 16 percent didn't shave, wax, or use electrolysis or laser methods

For women in their thirties and forties, about half removed some pubic hair but didn't go bare. Only about 9 percent of women in their thirties reported being bare much of the time over the past month, as did about 7 percent of women in their forties. We also found that bisexual women were more likely to go bare compared to straight or lesbian women. Women who were partnered were more likely to go bare at least some of the time, and those who were not sexually active generally didn't remove their pubic hair compared to other women.

What was particularly curious is that women who went bare some or much of the time had higher scores on measures of genital self-image and sexual function. This means that these women generally felt more positively about their genitals. They also generally experienced higher desire, higher arousal, and greater sexual satisfaction than women who didn't go bare. We're not really sure what this means. We find it difficult to believe that going bare automatically makes women like their genitals more or have better sex. We think it's more likely that women who are more into how their genitals look perhaps want to show them off, by taking it all off from time to time. Or maybe women who are highly into sex and who have arousing, satisfying, and perhaps more adventurous or experimental sex lives are more likely to be daring with their pubic hair, such as taking it all off. More research is needed to better understand how women's pubic hairstyles relate to the rest of their sex lives.

Perhaps the most important take-home message from this study is that—contrary to what we sometimes see in the media about there being one dominant pubic hairstyle for women—women do all kinds of different things to their pubic hair. Some do nothing. Some trim their hair. Others shave the sides off or shave it into shapes, such as a heart or a star. Some women shave or wax all of it off, or opt for electrolysis or laser methods to permanently reduce how much hair they have. As far as we're concerned, this is great news, as it means that there's no "standard" that women should feel pressured to live up to when it comes to their hair. Just as women's labia come in all sorts of shapes, sizes, and colors, pubic hairstyles are diverse, too.

We weren't the only ones that were excited about this finding from our study. After our study was published, numerous writers from women's magazines and blogs called us to ask about the study so they could share our results with their readers. Many of these writers thanked us for conducting the study and said that they, too, were tired of media articles that made it seem like every woman on the planet was as bare as a baby down there. Not that there's anything wrong with being bare—there's not, as far as we're concerned. But there's something really nice about finding out how individual we all are, and that more women than we may realize are bucking the so-called trends and doing whatever the heck they want down there.

WEARING YOUR HAIR

Now that we've talked about what other women do with their pubic hair, let's talk about you and your pubic hair. What follows are some basic tips for each type of style listed—just in case you're thinking about switching things up down there.

Going Natural

This is exactly what it sounds like. When you go natural, you don't trim, shave, wax, or engage in any kind of removal. Some women naturally have very little hair, whereas others boast a full natural "bush" that could stand up to even the wildest merkin on the market.

Advantages   No maintenance is required—just wash and air dry, and you're all set. Plus you may have hairs that are long enough to decorate with little ribbons or even braid. There are no side effects to going natural, and it's free! It's also coming back in style, albeit with a new name—the Retro Bush.

Disadvantages   You may find yourself in a bit of a pickle in swimsuit season; if you don't want the world to see your pubes, you may want to opt for a "boy short" swimsuit bottom. If you're okay flashing your hairs, like Miranda does in the *Sex and the City* movie, go for it! There's nothing wrong with going natural. Also, sexual partners of women with long or bushy pubic hair may find it more difficult to perform oral sex on them (then again, some people like a challenge, so this isn't a disadvantage for everyone).

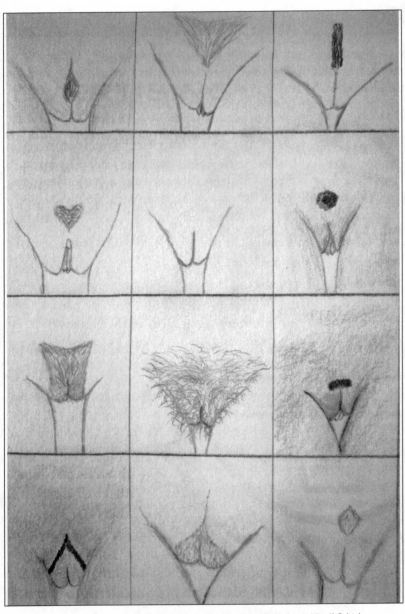

*Designing Women: Pubic Hair Patterns for All of Us (© Maleese Nicol' Schick.
See more of her work at www.Maleese.com.)*

Trimming

This is perhaps one of the most common forms of pubic hairstyling that men engage in, but it's also common among women. Tip: small scissors are often easier to maneuver than larger "craft" or kitchen scissors. Plus, no one wants pubes in kitchen scissors that may later be used on food items.

Advantages   Easy to do on your own and only needs to be done once every week or so to keep hair length in check. Trimming hairs can make it easier for partners to perform oral sex. There's also no risk of razor burn or chemical irritation and nothing to buy except for scissors (not a bad initial investment).

Disadvantages   Be careful not to cut yourself (rare, but it happens). There are also similar swimsuit considerations as noted in the "going natural" category.

Shaving

Many women choose to shave their pubic hair, especially if they prefer to not have pubic hair sticking out the sides of their underwear or bathing suits. You may get a closer shave using a double-edged razor blade. Some disposable razors come with soft lotion-strips to soften the skin post-shave. Shaving in the direction of hair growth can reduce the risk of razor burn (this is opposite to the direction that many women use to shave their legs).

Advantages   Inexpensive. You can do it yourself. Relatively easy to do once you get the hang of which direction to shave. Razors are also portable, so you can continue to shave while traveling.

Disadvantages   Hair can grow back quickly, which means you may be left with stubble or find yourself having to shave often (e.g., every day or so) to avoid stubble. Many women also find that they get razor burn or are prone to in-grown hairs as a result of shaving.

Depilatories

Depilatories are made of chemicals that remove hair. They come in different forms including gels, lotions, creams, and roll-on devices.

Not all depilatories are recommended for use in the genital area, so read any instructions or package inserts to make sure that you are using it correctly.

Advantages   Relatively inexpensive, you can do it yourself, and hair removal may be longer lasting than it is with shaving, leaving a smooth hair-free feeling.

Disadvantages   Some women are prone to irritation from chemicals commonly found in depilatories. You may want to do a skin test first (on another part of the body, such as your leg or inner arm), as is often recommended in the instructions that come with depilatories. Also, avoid using depilatories on skin that is inflamed or broken, such as if you have razor burn or sores.

Waxing

Pubic hair waxing has become increasingly popular over the past decade or so. Many full-service hair salons now offer bikini area waxing. There are also many waxing-specific salons, particularly in major cities such as New York (Completely Bare), San Francisco (Stript), and Chicago (The Waxing Room).

Advantages   Because waxing involves pulling the hair out at the root, it lasts longer than shaving or depilatories. The area that was waxed may feel smooth for one or more weeks following a treatment. There's also no risk of razor burn.

Disadvantages   The cost is moderate to expensive (the more hair removed, the more expensive). Also, the wax irritates some women's skin. Oh, and it can hurt like hell—especially the closer one gets to the inside parts of the outer labia. Plus, the terms can be confusing. For example, some salons describe a Brazilian wax as leaving a small "landing strip" of hair and a "Hollywood" as going completely bare. But when many other salons list "Brazilian," they're referring to removing every last hair. Our advice? Ask questions! Be specific with the aesthetician about what you do or do not want removed. (All the hair on top? What about the hair on your labia? What about the hair in your butt crack? Yes, some wax jobs go there . . . Be prepared to get awfully cozy with your aesthetician.) Finally, one often needs at least a couple weeks of hair growth in order to have hair that's long enough to wax off, so get ready to grow before you go.

VAJACIALS

A few years ago, Stript wax bar founder Katherine Goldman started offering vajacials in her Bay Area salons—essentially, treatments for women's vulvas about a week following their full Brazilian waxes.[13] The treatment is meant to care for women's skin and includes a warm wash, exfoliation, extractions (removal of ingrown hairs), and a mask that may include an antifreckle agent, an antibacterial agent, or a calming solution. The vajacial is finished off with a lightening treatment to even out skin tone. Last time we checked, it cost about $60. Though vajacials have gotten a lot of press (after all, they are yet another way for the vulva to become trendy!), we haven't seen any signs that would suggest they're sweeping the nation. Over the past few years, it's seemed as though inventing new words that start with VA and have something to do with women's sexy parts (e.g., vajazzling, vajacial, vatooing, vajayjay) has been enough to get a lot of traction in the blogosphere.

Sugaring

Sugaring is an all-natural method of hair removal. The "sugaring" paste is often made with ingredients such as sugar, lemon juice, and water (though salons may vary). Also called "sugar waxing," although technically, there shouldn't be any wax involved, at least not with the traditional Middle Eastern methods we are familiar with.

Advantages   A greater hair-covered area can be sugared off at once than with waxing. As such, sugaring may not take as long. Sugaring can be less painful than waxing (Debby tried this once years ago and concurs). You can also try mixing up your own sugar paste with recipes and instructions found online (you may want to try non-genital areas, such as your legs, before you experiment with sugaring your pubic hair).

Disadvantages   Sugaring hasn't taken off everywhere, so it can be difficult to find a salon that offers this service (some salons mix sugar with their wax and call it sugaring, but this is not the same). In salons, the cost is moderate to expensive, often close in price to waxing. Also, as with waxing, you often need at least a couple of weeks of hair growth in order to have enough length to sugar off.

Electrolysis

Electrolysis sounds more science fiction than salon, but it's been a common method of hair removal for years. It involves having a trained professional use a needle device (called an "epilator") or a tweezer epilator to send electric current to the hair root. It's meant to destroy the hair follicle so that hair won't grow back.

Advantages   When it works, it can result in permanent hair removal (or at least a reduction in the amount of hairs).

Disadvantages   Electrolysis can be expensive and require a series of treatments (home electrolysis kits are available but not often recommended). And it can be painful. Also, it sometimes doesn't work (the electric current may miss or not be enough), and the hair grows back. There are also risks of scarring, infection, and electric shock (the latter is uncommon but possible), and not all states require electrologists to be licensed.

Laser Hair Reduction

Laser hair reduction is one of the more recent innovations in hair removal. More doctor's offices now offer laser hair reduction. Before scheduling an appointment, you may want to ask who will be performing the treatment (if it's not the doctor, you should make sure that it will be performed by a technician who has specific training).

Advantages   Laser hair reduction has been shown to be more effective in reducing hair regrowth as compared to electrolysis. Newer lasers also make the treatment effective for a broader range of skin pigments and hair types than in years past. Often, several treatments are needed to reach one's desired results, so you should ask questions about roughly how many treatments are recommended, how you should prepare for the treatment, how much it will cost, what the technician's credentials are, and what you can expect as far as the treatment goes.

Disadvantages   Like electrolysis, not everyone who offers laser hair reduction is well-trained or experienced in it (again, ask before you schedule an appointment or go through with the procedure). Also, laser treatments can be quite painful, particularly the closer one gets to the outer labia. Ask about options for decreasing discomfort, such as the use of an anesthetic cream. Side effects are possible, including inflammation, hypopigmentation (areas of lightened skin), and hyperpigmentation (areas of darkened skin).

YOUR PERSONAL PUBIC STYLE: SOME THINGS TO CONSIDER

Given the many different options for one's pubic hair, there are several things that you may find helpful to consider as you choose your next pubic hairstyle or method of grooming:

- **Cost.** Try to select a method that you can afford to keep up. Some methods are particularly expensive. College women, for example, are more likely to shave than wax. Brazilian waxes, for many women, went by the wayside during the 2008 recession. And laser hair reduction? It's not unheard of for women to choose this longer-lasting, but more expensive, method of hair removal after they get their first job or a raise.

- **Convenience.** Ask yourself if this is a method that you can keep up on your own. If you're planning to go on a camping trip and don't expect to have access to regular showers, you may find it easier to either go totally natural or to do something longer lasting (like wax rather than shave) before your trip.
- **Upkeep.** Consider the upkeep. Trimming, for example, may only require weekly or biweekly attention. If you shave your pubic hair, you may find that you're smoothest with a daily or every-other-day shave. Electrolysis and laser hair reduction take less time and are done less often, but they do require one to make—and keep—appointments. How much time are you willing to put into your hair down there, and how often?
- **Your preference.** What pubic hairstyle helps you to feel confident? Sexy?
- **Your partner's preference.** What kind of pubic hairstyle turns your partner on? How do your preferences match up?
- **Hypersensitivities and allergic reactions.** Some women have more sensitive skin than others. If you're prone to razor burn, shaving may not be for you. And if you keep getting ingrown hairs, you may want to ask your healthcare provider about other options for grooming, such as laser hair reduction. Or just trim your hairs—if you're not getting them at the root, you'll be far less likely to encounter problems.
- **Steady hand.** The stories we could tell you of shaving and trimming gone wrong! Simply put, if you don't have a steady hand, or if you approach shaving or trimming your pubic hair with a great deal of anxiety, then leave it to the pros and have an aesthetician do your pubes for you. Either that or go completely natural. Years ago, Debby was at a vulvovaginal health conference and sat through a presentation that highlighted various hair removal injuries on women's vulvas, including many shaving strokes gone astray. Be careful out there!

- **When you're down with getting down.** If you're not a morning person, you might not want to grab a razor and hit up your downtown area until you are wide awake, alert, and have a steady hand. If your partner frequently intrudes on your showers, wait until you're alone to hop in the shower and shave your pubic hair into your preferred style—that way, your partner can't get in the way or make you nervous while you groom. If you're into waxing, you may want to schedule it for a time when you are not on your period, as some women feel more sensitive while menstruating.

- **Personal characteristics.** Believe it or not, your race/ethnicity may influence the best method of hair removal for you. In *The V Book: A Doctor's Guide to Complete Vulvovaginal Health,*[8] gynecologist Dr. Elizabeth Gunther Stewart describes how Caucasian women tend to have egg-shaped hair shafts, Asian and Native American women tend to have round hair shafts, and African American women tend to have elliptical-shaped hair shafts. As such, she says, different hair removal methods may work better for different women. She writes, for example, that African American women tend to be more prone to bumps from shaving but often have better results with laser hair reduction. Check out her book for more detailed information.

WHOSE HAIR IS IT, ANYWAY? HOW TO HAVE A PUBIC HAIR POWWOW WITH YOUR PARTNER

In her work as a sex columnist, Debby often hears from women and men who seek advice about how to talk with their partners about pubic hair. Sometimes the question comes from a woman or a man who wishes their partner would go bare, go natural, or do something fancy down there. Other times, the question is from someone who has long had one pubic hairstyle but now wants to change it up—they just aren't sure how their partner will react.

I feel that I am really lucky in that all of my sexual partners have been incredibly sex-positive and very educated and comfortable with my genitalia. I know from talking to my female friends that this is not always the case for many women, though, and often women are hurt or shamed by their partners' attitudes. I wish there was more information out there to help women realize that they should stand up for themselves and their bodies and not let sex-negative male partners shame them and make them feel insecure for the rest of their lives!
—ALYSSA, 24, New York

The key to good relationships and to good sex is communication, and the same is true for negotiating pubic hairstyles. If you'd like to have a pubic hair powwow with your partner, consider the following:

- Try to find a time when neither of you is distracted by anything else (e.g., television, studying, work, packing the kids' lunches). This could be while you're lying around on the sofa or when you're lying around post-sex.
- If you're the one who's thinking of changing your pubic hairstyle, and you worry that it will matter to your partner, bring it up. In your own words, say something about how you've been thinking about doing something different with your pubic hair and you'd like his or her opinion on the matter.
- If you're open to it, ask your partner if he or she would like to help out, such as by carefully shaving part of your hair, supportively cheering you on as you grow it out, or helping you create a pube-encil (see this chapter's activity).
- If you're hoping your partner will change his or her pubic hairstyle, start the conversation by saying something positive about your partner, such as how you find him or her sexy or attractive or that you love his or her body (maybe even his or her pubic hair specifically). Rather than saying that you don't like your partner's style and think he or she should change it, why not start from a more positive place? Suggest that an even sexier look might be fun (natural, trimmed, shaped like

ACTIVITY: DIY PUBE-ENCILS

If you'd like to customize your pubic hair into a shape, such as a heart or flower or the first letter of your or your partner's name, we invite you to consider making your own at-home pube-encil.

What You Will Need

- a washable marker
- scissors
- paper

1. Use your marker to draw your preferred shape on a piece of paper. You may want to hold up the piece of paper to your mons to make sure it's the size you want.
2. Cut out the shape by cutting along the lines that you have drawn.
3. Hold the shape up to your mons while you or a partner use a washable marker to trace around the shape. This will result in a shape drawn on to your vulvar skin. If you have questions or concerns about ink getting on your vulva, we recommend that you talk with a healthcare provider before trying this activity.
4. Trim the hairs outside the line, then shave or wax them off for total removal. This should result in a neat shape of pubic hair, which you can further trim or keep their natural length, depending on your preference for the finished look.

a lightning rod). Or say something like, "I thought I might enjoy/get turned on by grooming your pubic hair, if you'd let me." If your partner's not into your ideas, try not to take it personally. After all, it is his or her hair—you just get to play with it.

- If your partner wants you to change your pubic hairstyle and you're up for it, great! There are many ways to add variety to one's relationship or sex life, and this can be one of them. If you're not into your partner's suggestion, politely say so. You can always suggest an alternate style or ask if there are other things you can do, outside of the pubic hair realm, to please him or her.

• If you do decide to groom each other's pubic hair, be careful—especially with scissors or razors. When you shave yourself, it's easy to feel if you cut yourself or if you're shaving too hard. When you shave another person, it's not necessarily so clear, so be gentle. Also make sure to groom each other in a well-lit space—and not when you're drunk (save the wine or champagne for later on in your romantic interlude).

HAVE FUN WITH YOUR HAIR

There are many ways to enjoy your pubic hair. For example, you might

• **Check out a pubic hair dye.** Make sure to use one specially designed for the pubic area, such as Betty Beauty, and even then, make sure to patch test it away from your pubic area before using it there. Follow the instructions to reduce your risk of irritation.
• **Love your grays!** Even Samantha from *Sex and the City* went gray. If we live long enough, every single one of us will. Though it's a little unclear exactly when this happens for everyone, most people we've asked say that they get their first gray down there years after they go gray up top.
• **Give it a little tug.** Some women find it pleasurable to stroke or tug their pubic hair during masturbation, foreplay, while receiving oral sex, or during other types of sex.
• **Make it even prettier.** If you've got a lot of hair down there, why not go all out? Tie little bows around a few strands for a fancy look. Bare women shouldn't have all the fun, a la vajazzling. Besides, bows are way more affordable

than crystals or rhinestones. You can color coordinate your bows with your outfits. And if you've got a Pride party to go to, do them up in rainbow colors!

- **Get down with pube-encils.** Create your own stencils to more easily fashion your or your partner's pubic hair into the shape or letter of your choice.
- **Ask for help!** Many couples find it erotic to groom each other's pubic hair. As noted earlier, just go slowly, do it sober, and be careful. There's nothing sexy about accidentally nicking one's partner with a razor.

GIVING BIRTH BARE—OR WITH HAIR?

When Katherine Heigl's character gave birth in *Knocked Up*, many moviegoers noticed that her vulva was bare. For many women, this was surprising—after all, as one approaches her due date, the vulva may be more sensitive with increased blood flow to the pelvic area. Would one really want to risk the pain of getting waxed? And with a large late-third-trimester tummy, would one really be able to easily reach one's own vulva to shave?

Nurses, midwives, and OB/GYNs we spoke with had a different take on the matter. Some said that women in their labor and delivery rooms routinely had their vulvas shaved as a matter of course. Others noted that although pubic hair shaving had previously been common when women were admitted to the hospital to deliver, the practice had largely fallen out of favor where they work. At least one nurse said that it didn't matter, though, as many of her patients came to the hospital with their vulvas already bare from having waxed or shaved on their own.

Several studies have been conducted on the topic of shaving women's pubic hair for labor and delivery, with some finding that the practice has no impact on perineal infection or healing.[14] If there's no benefit to the practice, one can see why the practice has largely fallen

by the wayside. If you're pregnant, you might want to ask your OB/
GYN or midwife about his/her viewpoint on this matter and his/her
plans for your pubes. That way, you can also weigh in with your own
pubic preferences and ask the questions that matter to you.

TEST YOUR VQ

1. The least expensive (and safest) pubic hairstyle is
   a. going natural
   b. going totally bare
   c. shaving daily
   d. waxing monthly

2. The term for a "pubic wig" is
   a. mister
   b. muffin
   c. merkin
   d. muff

3. Which comedian famously "taught" Chelsea Handler about vaginal cleansing on TV?
   a. Sarah Silverman
   b. Joan Rivers
   c. Tina Fey
   d. Amy Sedaris

Answers

1. a
2. c
3. d

· 7 ·

Evulvalution

Vulva Culture

$\mathscr{T}$ake a moment to close your eyes and think of an artistic vulva image (or any vulva image really) made prior to the twentieth century. What have you come up with? With the exception of the few art history majors or vulva-art connoisseurs, it is likely that most of you did not have an image come to mind, unless perhaps you went looking for some of the images we mentioned earlier when discussing pubic hair.

Think back to some of the most famous female nudes throughout history. For us, some of the first images that come to mind are of Eve with her leaf strategically covering her genitals or Botticelli's fifteenth-century Venus with her hand (and hair) modestly hovering over her vulva. In contrast, consider some of the corresponding famous male nudes from similar time periods. Both Michelangelo's *David* and the *Creation of Adam* depict clear images of the penis. What about the vulva? Was it invisible until the creation of Internet pornography? Hardly. In this chapter we will explore the many ways in which vulvovaginal culture has manifested, from ancient mythology to masturbation workshops in New York City to contemporary online art-and-craft projects.

LET THERE BE VULVA! FROM THE BEGINNING

Vulvas have unarguably been around since the beginning of womankind, and vulva art goes back almost as far as herstory itself does. The first vulva representation available to our knowledge is that of the *Venus of Willendorf*, which dates back over twenty-five thousand to thirty thousand years to the Paleolithic era.[1,2] That's right—one of the oldest pieces of art in the world includes a representation of the vulva. She is a limestone statue discovered in the early twentieth century. By today's social standards, she would be considered obese and would likely be classified as unhealthy. However, researchers suspect that she was a symbol of beauty and fertility at the time she was created. The size of her body has received a great deal of discussion and debate, but there is less attention paid to her vulva. Some of the individuals who have mentioned her vulva have described it as everything from defined to pronounced to missing. To us, the appearance of her vulva is quite clear. In fact, if you examine an image of her closely (highly recommended), you can almost decipher both her inner and her outer labia. Not only did one of our first artistic representations of women have genitals, she had genitals with details! It seems as though she was a far cry from contemporary female figures (e.g., Barbie) in more ways than one.

I also want to say that since discovering how much I embrace my own vagina, enjoying the way it looks and feels, it has made me curious about other women. I am in love with my partner, who is male, and have considered myself heterosexual most of my life, but find myself curious about others' vaginas and find women's genitalia to be beautiful. I'm not sure if this is a sexual desire or not. I'm not sure I would call it an "orientation" because I am with a man, and I also don't want to appropriate that term, considering I have had none of the experience of a queer-identified person. But I do think that feeling comfortable and embracing my own body has led me to have new ideas about sexuality and the fluidity of desire. Deconstructing my own ideas about sex, bodies, and pleasure has opened my eyes to the possibility of new desires and attraction.

—JESSICA, 21, New York

The vulva of *Venus of Willendorf* was not the only ancient representation of women's genitals. Some of the earliest historical stories from

Mesopotamia contain positive references to women's genitals. There are both direct and indirect references to the vulva throughout songs and tales from the time. In translations of ancient poetry, both male and female genitals are referred to using positive words and metaphors. One poem even describes the vulva as "sweet like beer" (an association that we would expect to come from a college party, not ancient Mesopotamian literature).[3] In fact, the Mesopotamians felt so positively about women's genitals that they even had a goddess of the vulva, Nin-Imma. Nin-Imma was a fertility goddess whose name literally translates to "the goddess that creates everything."[3] Not a bad title if you ask us! The next time you are struggling for a positive term for your vulva, you may want to consider calling her your Nin-Imma. It doesn't have the ring of "vajayjay," but it does have a long history that may make it even more powerful than an Oprah-approved term.

RAISE A SKIRT TO GOOD FORTUNE

What do you call someone who flashes his/her genitals at you? Unless invited, that person is often called a flasher, and that behavior is often grounds for a call to the police. People tend to think of flashers as male, but what about female flashers? In one case in Madison, Wisconsin, female flashers were identified as the cause of a 2002 Halloween riot that resulted in broken windows, fires, and a general state of reckless chaos.[4]

Women flashing their various parts (breasts, vulvas, and bottoms) is encouraged at select times (e.g., Mardi Gras) and is the source of a very profitable business in some cases (e.g., *Girls Gone Wild*). In fact, the behavior is the basis for many strip clubs. So today, flashing your vulva would likely be viewed as a deviant or highly sexualized act. In ancient mythology, however, the stories were very different.

An investigation of the ancient mythology from several different continents reveals several surprisingly similar stories about anásyrma (flashing of the genitals or bottom). In Greek mythology, there is a tale of a mother named Demeter (the goddess of the harvest) who was left feeling lost and dismayed after her daughter Persephone (daughter of Zeus, the father of gods and men) was abducted to the underworld by Hades (the god of the underworld).[5] Demeter spiraled into what can likely be described as a deep depression as she searched for her daughter. While traveling despairingly in search for her abducted daughter, she met a woman by the name of Baubo. Stories about the way in which Demeter meets Baubo and their relationship vary. Regardless, one portion of the story remains the same in most versions of the tale: Baubo immediately lifted Demeter's spirits simply by lifting up her skirt. One Latin translation by Clemens states, "Having said so, she at once drew up her garments from down below and revealed to the sight the form of her privy parts; which Baubo tossing with hollow hand—for their appearance was puerile—strikes, handles caressingly."[6]

To us, it sounds as though she also masturbated when she lifted up her skirt. We have also heard that she was a postmenopausal woman who was masturbating, which would be a wonderful celebration of sexual pleasure for all ages! Unfortunately, we were unable to find any historians who explicitly support (or mention) her masturbation in this context. There is, however, a consensus on the positive impact Baubo's vulva-flashing has on Demeter, who immediately cheered and drank the potion that was offered to her.[6] That one simple act is said to have ended a long sorrowful journey for Demeter. In celebration of that story, ancient statues of Baubo were carved and have been located in numerous places throughout Europe. Many statues represent Baubo as two legs with a large triangle for a face and a vulva in place of her chin. Other figurines emphasize a pronounced vulva, representing the importance of the vulva in ancient Greek mythology and art.

The story of Baubo in Greek mythology has a surprising number of similarities with ancient tales from both Egypt and Japan. According to Japanese mythology, the sun goddess Amaterasu was tortured by her brother, the wind-god Susanowo.[5] While this starts as simple brother/sister teasing, it escalates and results in the death of one of her maids. This frightens her (as it would anybody), and she decides to hide in the rocks and refuses to come out despite pleas from numerous gods and goddesses. After multiple attempts from many to get her out of her hiding spot, Uzume, the Dread Female of Heaven, revealed her genitals to Amaterasu. This action caused eight hundred gods and goddesses to break out into a laughter so deep that it caused the land to shake. Amaterasu was surprised by the laughter, assuming that everyone would be in profound sorrow waiting for her to come out of her hiding spot. For the first time since going into hiding from her brother, Amaterasu left her cave, bringing light back to the world.

Similar to the story of Amaterasu in Japanese mythology and Baubo in Greek mythology is the story of Ra in Egyptian mythology. This Egyptian tale takes place during a time of turbulence between gods and begins when a god by the name of Ra is insulted. He was evidently very upset by this insult and proceeded to sulk, refusing to speak to anyone.[5] As with Demeter, no one was able to cheer him until a goddess exposed her private parts to him. And as in the story of Baubo, this caused him to laugh, ending his desolate emotional state. This story is honored during the celebration of Bast, one of the most popular during its time in Egypt. During the celebration, women traveled on barges and shouted crude insults to those onshore, often exposing their vulvas as they did. Thus, as with the Baubo figurines, the commemoration of these stories demonstrates how celebrated the skirt-lifters once were.

To this date, there remains an intellectual debate between historians about *why* lifting a skirt and exposing genitals would result in so much laughter (apparently they don't think vulvas are as humorous as we do—see the "Vulvas Are Funny" sidebar).

It has been suggested that the laughter was a result of the surprise/shock of seeing a(nother) woman's genitals. It is also possible that what was considered humorous at the time may have been quite different than what is today, and that people were amused by the degradation of others for their amusement. If this is the case, then the stories indicate that these women/goddesses were actually humiliated by raising their skirts. While this is possible, it seems less likely, given that the skirt-lifting was done of their own free will.

VULVAS ARE FUNNY: A PERSONAL ANECDOTE

After sitting quite nicely through a friendly (yet somewhat formal) dinner where we somehow managed to keep the conversation off of vulvas for at least two straight hours (back pat), we headed over to a comedy club. At one point, the comedian made a comment about vulvas that Debby felt was a bit vagina-negative. It's not clear whether the quiet formality of the night overtook Debby or whether that glass of wine had just taken its toll, but in an effort to counter his comment, Debby yelled out, "But we love vulvas!" It worked. The comedian stopped his monologue, asked her what she said, and she repeated it, which got them into a brief conversation about vulvas. Soon enough, he was working vulva love into his stand-up routine. Although we like to think that the vulva awareness helped everyone that night, we felt particularly inspired by a joyful conclusion. Not only are vulvas powerful and feminist and shocking—they can also be funny.

Alternatively, pulling from several other lines throughout the ancient texts, theorists suggest that it is the unusual appearance of the skirt-lifters' vulvas that triggered the laughter.[6] For instance, authors point to a line about Baubo's genitalia that states that it is similar to that of a little boy who is flaccid and without hair. Still, some historical theorists suggest that Demeter's laughter is caused by the fact that Baubo shaves her pubic hair,[7] while others suggest that she has an enlarged clitoris and is perhaps intersex.[6] We don't have the answer but do think it is interesting that a modern interpretation of this ancient, joyous tale of the vulva has been changed into a story about the mockery of deviant genitalia and/or the humiliation of the women who show it.

VULVAS ON DISPLAY

Figurines of Baubo were not the only ancient figurines with prominent vulvas found throughout Europe. Have you ever approached someone's home or a building and stopped to wonder whether it would result in enhanced fertility, protection against evil, or warnings against lustful behavior? It is unlikely. These days, few modern buildings are adorned with symbolic carvings or figurines, and even fewer of these figurines have large, pronounced vulvas. Conversely, figurines designed for this exact purpose have been located throughout Ireland and Spain. Dated back to approximately the eleventh century, these figurines were not so different from some of the Baubo carvings. The figurines had large, round heads and small, undefined torsos with breasts and two thin legs spread wide open (not unlike the lithotomy position you climb into at your gynecologist's office) with large, open vulvas/vaginas as the central focal point. There are at least sixty-five buildings with these figurines in Ireland alone.[8]

The name of the figurines, sheela-na-gigs, is about as unclear as their purpose. While some have claimed that the name translates to "immodest woman," others believe that it is simply a name for the crouched position of the sheela-na-gigs. Like the name, people have speculated that sheela-na-gigs are everything from gargoyles that protect buildings to evil spirits to warnings against immodesty to representations of goddesses.[8] We may never be sure what the meaning of sheela-na-gig is (although our vote is for the goddess) but we do know that we like the idea of hanging a vulva statue outside our door to welcome guests. We are particularly fond of this idea for gynecologists' offices.

SOCIAL CUNTSRUCTIONS

What are the exterior parts of women's genitals called? Hopefully, at this point in the book you guessed "vulva." If you did, you're correct. Okay, now hop into an intellectual time machine and go back to before the fourteenth century. Same question: what do you call women's genitals? Sure, you can still use the terms "vulva" or "genitals," but now you have another option. You can also use the term "cunt"! That's right, once upon a time, the term was not insulting or derogatory; it was simply another term used to refer to women's genitals. The name is believed to have stemmed from the Asian goddess Cunti (knowing what you now know about the relationship between goddesses and the vulva, we hope that this is not as difficult to believe as it once was). Therefore, it is quite possible that the origin of the word was positive and powerful.

We really need a good word that means "vulva, labia, vagina, and clitoris."
A positive word. People get snarky and mean about women who say "vagina"
when they mean the genital area as a whole, but I think that is a load of crap.
People often use a part to represent the whole, especially when there is no good
word for the whole. Don't be a douche. Most of the women doing that know
perfectly well what the word vagina really means.

—PEGGY, 24, Minnesota

One of the first-documented uses of the word "cunt" was found on a street sign from the Middle Ages in England. The name of the street was Gropecunt Lane because of the purpose of the street at the time.[9] In the same way that some cities use grids systems, they used to name streets for the purposes they served. So the street received its name for the number of prostitutes who worked there. There were several other streets with similar names throughout Europe. Can you imagine proposing that street name at your local community board meeting today? Forget the meaning, the word "cunt" would probably send everyone into a frenzy. Well, it was apparently just fine until approximately the seventeenth century when the word was deemed obscene and inappropriate.[10] Even today, in contemporary times, many people feel that cunt is a negative word. (And in all fairness, it is often used in a derogatory way, so that doesn't exactly help things.) Some feminist activists hope to reclaim the word and the power behind it, returning it to its positive place. Vanessa tried to be a part of this cunt-positive movement in graduate school. It's tricky, though, as, "thank you" is often not the automatic retort to being called a cunt. However, we recommend giving it a try!

THE STORY OF SARAH BAARTMAN

In the early nineteenth century, a few centuries after "cunt" went out of style, the vulva had another major blow to its self-esteem. In 1825, a woman by the name of Sarah Baartman was a slave in Capetown, Africa. Originally Khoisan, the family she worked for encouraged her to travel to England under the false guise that it would lead to her emancipation and corresponding riches.[11] To her surprise and horror, freedom was a far cry from what she was forced to endure throughout her life and after her death. She shared the distinctive feature common to many Khoisan women called steatopygia, which was characterized by protruding buttocks and portly thighs. In order to display these "distinctive" features, all of her clothing was taken from her, and she was paraded around stages/cages as a spectacle for the fine men and women of England to gawk at. While her "large protruding buttocks" were her primary claim to "fame," you can find extensive descriptions about her genitalia if you dig through the history books a bit deeper. She was poked and prodded while onstage in order to display her vulva to crowds of judgmental onlookers.[12]

The English men and women of the time gave Ms. Baartman the nickname of Venus Hottentot and her long, flowing inner labia received the most scrutiny of all. Thus, inner labia that were long or dark in color became labeled as "other," as "deviant," and as "improper." After her death, her genitals were pickled and placed in a museum for years to shame her and any onlookers who may have had similar genitals hiding underneath their petticoats. (Sadly, the genitals of some African men were also kept in jars by Westerners who saw these individuals as more curiosities than living, breathing humans of equal value.)

FREUD'S PSYCHO-GENITAL-ICAL ANALYSIS

Sigmund Freud, the founder of psychoanalytic theory in the early twentieth century, is often considered controversial by contemporary psychologists. However, one thing can be said for certain about Freud: he put a lot of thought into the importance of genitals (or lack thereof). In fact, he believed that the genitals played a key role in the psychosexual development of both males and females. He believed that it was a psychologically momentous event for young boys or girls to see the genitals of someone of the opposite sex for the first time.[13] For young girls, the scene would go something like this: newly out of diapers (somewhere between 3.5 and 6 years old), she is sitting around minding her own business when she suddenly notices a penis. She looks down between her legs to find that she is without such a bulge and becomes overtaken with envy of the long schlong. Why? Well, the answer is simple. According to Freud, the sight of a penis leads to the realization that she will be unable to sexually satisfy her mother. Yep, her mother. So, she develops a desire for her father, and the soap opera plotline thickens. This, of course, is not an entirely conscious process, making it a tricky theory to test.

What do we think about penis envy, you ask? We say penis envy, schmenis envy. Not to hate on male genitals (we want men to feel good about themselves, too!), but vulvas have distinct advantages:

1. With a vulva, you never have to worry about covering your excitement with a book when called to the front of the classroom.
2. You always have the option to sit in the privacy of your own bathroom stall.
3. Your genitals have been compared to flowers and fruit.
4. You have your own private pleasure button.

That's not to say that there aren't advantages to having a penis, either. Some men play with their genitals to the point that they call it penis "puppetry." And they can pee pretty much anywhere without having to worry about sitting down. To the extent that this makes lines for men's public restrooms that much shorter certainly creates envy in many women. But still, we're happy with what we have, and we hope that men are happy with their parts, too.

Speaking of their parts—if Freud thought that women had penis envy, does that mean that he thought males must have penis pride? Not quite. Let's go back to our stage. A little boy in the same age range is again none the wiser when—BAM!—he is confronted with a vulva. Instead of being in awe of the beauty of the vulva or even thankful for his own little package, he is psychosexually traumatized by the event. That's right; Freud proposes that his reaction is not actually one of appreciation but one of fear. To him, the vulva looks like a slit where a penis used to be, and he concludes that the woman (likely his mom) must have had a penis at one time that has since been removed. This leads to what Freud terms "castration anxiety" that someone will slice off his penis (although penectomy anxiety would be a better term because castration implies that only the testicles have been removed). How would this happen, you ask? As far as we know, Freud does not exactly specify how men fear this will happen.

Do Vaginas Have Teeth?

Freud's non-specificity about castration anxiety would not be particularly noteworthy if it was not for the obvious omission of famous folklore that warned of a toothed-vagina. This belief is titled "vagina dentata" and has a long history from early mythology to contemporary stories in which men's penises are severed after inserting them (often forcefully) into women's vaginas. Depending on who tells or interprets the stories, they can be viewed as forewarnings of the dangers of women to men or a forewarning to men about the dangers of forcing oneself on a woman. Either way, according to Freud, seeing a vulva leads to castration anxiety in males. As such, although we wouldn't describe it as the most positive of theories about the vulva, it did bring genital issues back up for discussion.

YOU SAY LILY, I SAY LABIA

If you ever mention vulva art to anyone who knows art, one of the first artists they are likely to mention is Georgia O'Keeffe. She was born into a large family in the late nineteeth century on a farm in Wisconsin. Later in life, she attended the University of Virginia and then Columbia University for art classes, where some of her later art was inspired.[14] During this time, she also became involved with the National Women's Party, an organization formed to advance the women's suffrage movement. In 1924, she exhibited her first now-famous large still–life floral paintings.[14] The similarity of the appearance of her flowers to vulvas in these famous still–life paintings is unmistakable. Still, she denied that the paintings were intended to represent anything other than flowers. When asked about it, she once said "when you took time to really notice my flower you hung all your associations with flowers on my flower, and you think and see of the flower—and I don't."[15] In other words, she attributes any aesthetic similarities between her paintings and women's genitals to the natural resemblance of flowers to vulvas, as opposed to the intentional imitation many people had assumed. Because her initial art exhibits coincided with Freud's early publications on psychoanalytic theory, the meanings of the flowers were further deconstructed by their relationship to women's genitals. Whether or not the flowers' resemblance to women's genitals was intentional is unclear. Though, one thing we can be certain of is that the paintings remain one of the most popular representations of vulvas in history, even if unintentionally.

I wish women knew there is no one right model for how female genitals are supposed to look. Small is not better than large, "tidy" is not better than loose and floppy. They all are capable of doing their jobs—feeling good, giving pleasure, containing, taking in, protecting, accommodating, opening to give birth. Female genitalia are gorgeous, awe-inspiring, powerful, sensitive, diverse, vulnerable, and nothing to be ashamed of. Looking at female genitalia is like looking at a garden—tulips or freesias are not better than daffodils or tiger lilies.
—BARBARA, 61, California

The relationship between Georgia O'Keeffe, art, and vulvas does not end with her artistic representations of flowers. She was also the most contemporary woman to be seated at the table for *The Dinner*

Party.[16] This installation by Judy Chicago depicts 1,038 women who have made substantial contributions throughout time. Chicago's piece was inspired by the belief that much of art was designed based on history, and she wanted to create an artistic piece that represented herstory instead. With a great deal of help from other women over several years, she created a vulvastic piece of art with thirty-nine powerful and influential women sitting around a dinner table (hence the name).

"Why so vulvastic," you ask? First, the dinner table was shaped like a triangle with three equal sides. For many people, the triangle is evocative of the vulva (in particular, the mons). The real kicker comes from the way that the women at the table were represented. She could have created wax figures or paintings, but instead—as alluded to earlier in the pubic hair chapter—Chicago decided to pay homage to each woman with a beautiful and unique vulva-like place setting. There were also more than nine hundred names of other women who united these individuals or were worth recognizing in some way. As far as we're concerned, beautiful + unique + female unity + vulva = vulvastic! The dinner party is still on display and can be visited at the Brooklyn Museum in the Elizabeth A. Sackler Center for Feminist Art. It is a must-see on any vulva adventurer's scavenger-hunt list.[16]

VULVACTIVISM

You may be thinking that Judy Chicago was pretty brave to bring vulvas to public awareness. She was, but she certainly was not the only one. In fact, the 1970s were a pretty revolutionary time for the vulva and vagina. The 1960s–1970s were the decades of vulva awakening and awareness. Women from around the United States began to come together to talk about their lives and roles as women in groups that were called consciousness-raising groups. It was an important time for feminism, and these women did some pretty kick-ass things. In some of the groups, the women would discuss their bodies and would become frustrated by how little they knew about them. They decided that the best way to take control over their bodies and sexualities was to take matters into their own hands (literally).

V-CRAFT: VULVA *MOLDEL*:
MAKING YOUR VERY OWN VULVA ART

What You Will Need

- alginate
- water
- a large, shallow bowl or medium-sized pan/tin
- plastic gloves
- plastic wrap (optional)
- Vaseline (optional)
- a large plastic bag (large trash bags work well)
- a comfortable place to sit sans pants for several minutes
- a book full of creative ideas for the vulva mold (check!)

Steps

1. Do you want to be a vulva moldel? There are probably lots of ways to go about this, but this is one way we recommend! You actually only need a few ingredients to create a vulva mold, and most of these can probably be found around the house. The only ingredient that you may not have is alginate. You can probably use several different things to make a cast, but we recommend alginate because that is what the artists we talked to recommend. Fortunately, purchasing alginate should not be a terribly difficult or expensive process. If they do not have it at your local arts-and-crafts store, you can find it for sale on numerous web sites. You don't need a lot of alginate for a single mold, so no need to order a bulk size (unless you are having a vulva casting party!). When purchasing online, you may want to consider contacting the seller ahead of time to ask how much water he/she recommends adding to the alginate because it may vary by seller. However many cups of water it takes for you to completely submerge your vulva is probably about the amount of alginate you should order for a single vulva mold.

2. First things first, alginate can be messy and tricky to clean. You will want to cover your workspace with a non-porous material. Some extra trash bags or plastic shopping bags should do the trick! Cover all the areas of your home/clothing that you want to protect, as you would do with any other art project.

3. Once you have acquired some alginate and set up your workspace, the rest is easy. First, you have to decide how comfortable you are with the alginate touching your skin. It is possible that you may be allergic. If you decide to place it directly on your skin, it is a good idea to test it on your inner labia (they may be more sensitive than your other skin) at least twenty-four hours in advance. In addition to being sensitive or allergic, if you apply the alginate directly to your skin, you risk pulling out some very sensitive hairs down there. It may work for shorter hair if covered in Vaseline or another protective agent, but it is risky. Also, we don't recommend putting it directly on your genitals if you have any cuts, sores, or scrapes. To be on the safe side, we recommend wrapping your genitals in plastic wrap or other material (e.g., latex for the allergy-free) that you feel comfortable placing on your genitals. Take some time with this. The more detailed your wrapping job, the more detailed your mold will be.

4. Once you have made sure that your genitals are ready to mold, pour the appropriate amount of alginate into a separate container (not the mixing/molding bowl), and fluff it with your hands until you have gotten out all of the lumps. Next, measure the appropriate amount of water. Every alginate is different, so be sure to follow the directions you were provided. Pour the water into the molding container, followed by the alginate. *Quickly* squeeze the batter through your fingers to smooth it as best you can.

5. Once the batter is mixed, you have to continue to move very quickly because alginate takes under ten minutes to dry. So place the molding tray on a pre-covered chair or floor, and position yourself strategically above it. Dip in as much of your genitals as you want included in the mold. Sit very still.

> 6. Approximately ten minutes later, the mold should have hardened. Carefully remove your genitals from the solution and . . . voila! Enjoy the vulvastic mold you just created!
> 7. The options are endless. You can paint it and put it on your wall (for the brave and bold) or in a drawer (for the brave and discreet). Consider adding some chocolate for a delicious, sexy treat or some soap for some good clean fun. Enjoy!
>
> Interested but sound a little too complicated? You may want to consider purchasing a kit from an online retailer. We suggest the one from holisticwisdom.com.

During some of these parties, the women would gather together with speculums to look inside and learn all about their own vulvas, vaginas, and cervixes. We were not around during the time of these parties, so we can only imagine how liberating they must have felt for the women participants. Just think about how wonderful it would be to change your associations with speculums from the fear and discomfort you feel at the gynecologist's office (if you are like many women) to feelings of excitement, curiosity, and sisterhood. Even if you are not interested in starting your own speculum party, you may be interested in purchasing one to learn all about the ins and outs of your vulva.

Betty Dodson

Many women in the United States attended and led consciousness-raising groups during the 1970s. One well-known group leader was Betty Dodson, a foremother in the genital advocacy movement. She has written several books (including *Sex for One: The Joy of Selfloving* and *Orgasms for Two: The Joy of Partnersex*) that tell of her plight for genital-diversity awareness.[17] She came to accept her genitals only after looking over a series of "beaver shots" that depicted a normal range of genital images (these were obviously not today's magazines—see Chapter 4: How Do I Look? for more information).

Inspired by the beauty of the natural diversity of women's genitals, she took photos of numerous courageous women's vulvas. Betty showed these pictures at a National Organization for Women conference in 1973 in a presentation titled "Creating a Genital Aesthetic." For many women, this was the first time that they had ever seen genital images, and she writes about how shocked many of the women were to see these images.[17] After the picture show was finished, she was met with a resounding applause. Since then, she has continued to work tirelessly advocating for genital awareness and acceptance. One of the things she has become famous for are her masturbation workshops. Similar to speculum parties, Betty's masturbation workshops focused on helping women to learn about their own bodies in order to enrich their potential for sexual pleasure and orgasm. She found that one of women's biggest barriers to sexual pleasure was their anxiety about the appearance of their genitals. As such, in the masturbation circles, she would ask the women to go around and discuss these concerns honestly and openly with one another. Later in the session, they would have a genital show-and-tell, and some even had a genital portrait taken. It allowed the women to learn that their genitals were natural, normal, and beautiful. Betty has written extensively and taped several videos on this exact topic, which are now available on DVD. In our experience showing these films to women and men, we've found that more people come to appreciate their genitals—and learn a few tips for sexual pleasure as well.

Annie Sprinkle

Betty Dodson was not the only genital activist (or in her words, "vulvactionist") who promoted genital acceptance through art. Annie Sprinkle has advocated similarly powerful genital messages. If the name itself doesn't make you smile, maybe her work will. Sprinkle is a former sex worker/porn-star extraordinaire and a foremother in sex-positive feminism who continues to work as an activist and artist.[18] She has conducted a variety of art shows and engaged in numerous activist projects meant to disrupt the way that we think about women's sexualized bodies. At one point in her earlier career, she created a small business with a close friend selling locks of pubic hair, vials of urine, and used panties. Does this sound like a list of things that you would dread confronting in a shared bathroom? Probably—but that's exactly her point! They are all part of natural body functions and experiences and what it means to be human. And yet many of us feel repelled by these very things.

It makes us think of that book *Everyone Poops*.[19] Well, everyone urinates and pretty much everyone grows pubic hair and wears panties (at least some of the time). Yet, for some reason, we are embarrassed or ashamed about these things. Annie's business venture pointed out that pubic hair and excretory functions are not only natural, but they can also be sexy! How great is that?! This is not her only urine venture, either. She would always end one totally amazing performance-art piece by standing upside-down and urinating a bright golden firework of a finale.[18] We never had a chance to attend the show, but we would put money on the fact that her audiences never left pissed (we couldn't resist).

There are almost too many amazing Annie Sprinkle performance-art shows and presentations to count. However, one of the performance-art pieces of particular relevance to the vulva was her show "Post-Porn Modernist."[18] Performed throughout the early 1990s, "Post-Porn Modernist" featured a segment brilliantly titled "The Public Cervix Announcement," where she would unabashedly show her cervix to the audience members. She would start by douching, inserting a speculum into her vagina, and then asking the audience members to line up to view her cervix. Audience members who did were handed a flashlight and encouraged to ask questions. Sprinkle gave the audience three reasons why she thought it was important to show her cervix:[18, 20]

> Reason number one: a cervix is such a beautiful thing and most people go through their whole lives and never get to see one. I'm really proud of mine, and I'd like to give that opportunity

to anyone who'd like to have it. Reason number two is, I find it's a lot of fun to show my cervix in little groups like this. And reason number three is, I want to prove to some of the guys out there that there are absolutely no teeth inside there.

Not only does Sprinkle try to remind the audience that the vulva and vagina are places of beauty and mystery, she also reassures the audience that they can be both safe and fun. Unfortunately, she no longer performs this particular performance-art piece, but she remains one of the foremothers of the sex-positive movement. For more about Sprinkle, check out our Resources section.

And Then There Was Eve

The 1960s and 1970s were a powerful time for the vulva-activism movement. Women from across the United States were uniting to discuss and discover their vulvas. Then, something happened. Maybe it was the new wave of feminism. Maybe it was everyone's obsession with exercise (and body size) in the 1980s. However, feminist-consciousness groups came to a halt (not a screeching one—they still exist but are fewer and farther between) and with them, many women's interest in discovering and understanding their bodies—or at least their vulvas. Sure, women like Betty and Annie persisted in their work, but overall, people stopped talking about vulvas, vaginas, cunts, and twats. For some time, vulvas and vaginas went underground and were rarely talked about in any mainstream way.

And then there was Eve.

In 1996, Eve Ensler came out with the now-infamous play, *The Vagina Monologues*. Based on interviews with approximately two hundred women, the play highlights a series of topics related to women's vulvas and vaginas including menstruation, vaginal smell, taste, rape, sexual exploration, oppression, vaginal birth, pleasure, and the word "cunt."[21] The play took off and became wildly popular. Over a period of years, celebrities such as Oprah Winfrey, Jane Fonda, Julia Stiles, and

FEMALE GENITAL CUTTING

We would be remiss if we didn't mention female genital-cutting practices, sometimes described as "female genital mutilation (FGM)" or "female genital circumcision," depending on one's perspective. Although many girls and women have suffered from the physical consequences or even died as a result of genital-cutting practices, the term FGM is offensive to many girls and women who have been circumcised and feel more beautiful or womanly as a result of the procedure. While we don't like the idea of people cutting women's vulvas—especially when they are children and may not be able to consent to the procedure or understand the potential for health complications—we also don't like the idea of making women feel badly for something (like having been circumcised) that is a common part of their culture, which has happened to them (perhaps not by choice) and which they may embrace.

In fact, we're far from the only feminists to face such a crisis of how to respond to female genital-cutting practices and even how to talk about them. Millions of pages have been written about the practice, and we certainly can't do the cultural, sexual health, and very personal features of these practices justice in this book. But we do want to provide some basic information and suggest resources for more information in what we feel is culturally sensitive advocacy.

What It Entails

There are several different types of female genital-circumcision practices. In a 1994 article published in the *New England Journal of Medicine*, Dr. Nahid Toubia grouped these practices into four types[22]:

- Type 1 clitoridectomy refers to removal of part or all of the clitoris; also commonly known as the "Sunna circumcision."
- Type 2 clitoridectomy refers to the excision of the clitoris as well as part of the labia minora. The urethra and vaginal opening remain visible and accessible.
- Type 3 may be referred to as an "intermediate" infibulation. It involves removal of the clitoris and labia minora and the stitching

together of the labia majora, leaving a moderate-sized opening for urine, menstrual blood, and vaginal discharge to leave the body.
- Type 4, also called total infibulation, is a more extreme version of infibulation in that only a small opening is left for fluids to leave the body.

Because female genital-circumcision procedures are typically carried out by laypersons (often female elders in a community), there is wide variation in the type and amount of cutting, so these are only general guidelines. We would never want this to happen to us, but then again, we both grew up in cultures in which these practices are largely unheard of and doctors are not allowed to perform them.

Being "outsiders" to this practice presents specific challenges in how to respond to it. Some people feel that it's the work of feminism to oppose practices worldwide that are harmful to women. Others feel that it's quite patriarchal for (largely) Western women to be so critical of cultural practices that they are not a part of and can't ever truly understand—perhaps particularly when many Western women willingly engage in all sorts of body cutting in their own quest for perfection, beauty, or symmetry (e.g., breast-implant surgeries, elective female-genital surgeries such as labiaplasty, liposuction, etc.).

What We Do Know Is This

- We love vulvas as they are and hope that one day these practices go away. However, we feel that changing this is best done in a culturally sensitive way. The V-Day organization, for example, has a long history of supporting a safe house in Kenya that assists young women who wish to escape this practice and instead live at the safe house and receive education. To learn more about how you can support this kind of work, visit VDay.org.
- Women from cultures or countries where these practices are common should not be asked about the state of their genitals except by people whose business it is to know, such as their healthcare providers, partners, or midwives. We know of some African women who, for example, have been asked by complete

strangers if they have "been mutilated." Would you want a stranger asking you about your genitals?
- Although it's commonly said that women who have experienced genital cutting cannot and do not experience sexual pleasure, this is not always the case. Research has found that many women who have experienced genital cutting are indeed able to experience sexual pleasure and orgasm, even if their genitals are not intact.
- Women who have had this done should not be made to feel ugly or damaged or "mutilated." We are all beautiful and valuable regardless of what has been done to our genitals, whether by choice, cultural pressure, or force.

For more information about female genital-cutting practices, visit VDay.org or the World Health Organization (who.org).

Rosie Perez performed the monologues for various shows. It made the vagina a household name and opened up conversations around many topics that were previously considered too taboo to discuss. The show has been translated into numerous languages and continues to be performed across the globe (Debby has performed in local productions of *The Vagina Monologues* several times). If you are interested in seeing the show or being a part of it, many college campuses continue to perform the show annually.

Although *The Vagina Monologues* was originally intended as a celebration of the vagina and women, it is now often performed to support V-Day: A Global Movement to End Violence against Women and Girls. While there are few people who would not applaud the promotion of anti-violence efforts, some critics, such as Betty Dodson, are less positive about the association between violence and the vagina.[23] Others fault the play (which was eventually made into an HBO special) for failing to include pictures of vulvas/vaginas. Still others critique the use of the term "vagina" when the play is predominantly about the "vulva," a term which, according to critics, may have become popularized if used in the play.[23] In her defense, Eve is said to have believed that the title would have been confusing to those who were not aware of the meaning of the word "vulva." It will never be known whether *The Vulva Monologues* would have flopped or whether it would have made "vulva" a household name, but we do know that *The Vagina Monologues* got people talking about a subject that they may not have discussed without the play. In fact, it is unlikely that this book would have been possible without her work. For many reasons, including this one, we are incredibly thankful for Eve Ensler and her groundbreaking work—the woman who got the word "vagina" on marquees worldwide, encouraged audiences to chant the word "cunt," and inspired women to honor the "vagina warriors" in their lives.

THE GOOD, THE BAD, AND THE FAMOUS.COM

Fifteen years ago, the terms "Google," "poke," "tweet," and "sext" were probably meaningless to you. You had to arrange to meet friends ahead of time, answering machines were used to screen calls, and cameras (with film!) were used to take pictures that you had to wait a minimum of an hour to see. Recent technological inventions have changed the way we think, feel, and talk about the vulva. Our ability to capture a picture at a moment's notice has made panty-less celebrities who exit their limos one of the most commonly discussed vulva-related conversations. Sure, this is probably not a new phenomenon. If you think about it, one of the most famous pictures of any celebrity is the image of Marilyn Monroe in that flowing white halter dress taken from *The Seven Year Itch* where she appears to be trying to hide her genitalia (or at least her underwear) as the wind shoots her skirt up from below.

Modern-day upskirt shots are different and so is the way that we talk about them. Within the past few years, several of today's hottest celebrities have found themselves in panty-less predicaments. They go out one lovely evening donning a fetching mini-skirt or dress. Presumably, the dress is oftentimes not only short but quite tight. In fact, it is likely too tight to wear with panties (sorry—this is beginning to sound like the beginning of a bad porn). Not wanting to be caught on film with panty lines (or perhaps to feel super sexy or just plain comfortable), they leave their panties at home and cross their fingers/legs that no sneaky photographer has decided to wear shoes with mirrors on the tops that evening.

Fortunately, while no celebrity to our knowledge has fallen victim to mirrored shoes, they have been caught by a similarly sneaky move. When crouched at the right angle, photographers can snap a picture up the celebrity's skirt as she steps out of her car. When they do, do the photographers say, "Oops, got the vulva," and then quietly delete the photo? No. There is money to be made from a picture of a celebrity without underwear. Consequently, a number of these photos have wound up on the Internet.

So far, this story is understandable to us. The celebrity left the house likely hoping that no one would be the wiser about her undergarments (or lack thereof). The term "money shot" is not lost on the photographer, and he/she publishes the picture for financial gain. Are we fans of this? No. But we understand how it happens. Where we feel the story gets interesting is in the public's reaction to the pictures. Are we, the public, shocked and appalled that the photographer would snap a private picture without the celebrity's permission and put it on the Internet for all to see? Perhaps some are, but the public's outrage is usually directed toward the female celebrity. She is vilified for daring to leave the house without the "proper" undergarments. Even though seemingly accidental, these celebrities are deemed promiscuous even though the picture was entirely unrelated to their sexual behavior. Not only that, but her vulva becomes the easy target of criticism by commenters who apply a mob mentality to her most private parts. We've read anonymous comments that not only shame these women for leaving their homes without underwear, but also attempt to shame them for the way their genitals look. It's particularly upsetting to us when anonymous commenters describe women's vulvas as looking "used up" or "slutty." Since when can a woman's genitals tell you anything about her sexual behavior?

We felt that one ex–teen star's comment on a recent talk show summed up these comments nicely. Let's call her Brenda. During Brenda's teen stardom, she was widely known for being rebellious and temperamental. When Brenda was asked about her teenage rebellions, she said something along the lines of "at least I always wore panties." As though showing your vulva (accidentally) can be the worst thing that a girl can do! It is no wonder women feel so uncomfortable showing their vulvas to their doctors or loved ones. These are clearly not the messages passed down from our sex-positive foremothers.

The disparaging comments made about celebrities' vulvas are particularly difficult for us to digest. When researching some of these pictures and their corresponding comments, we noticed that people had taken the opportunity to insult the appearance of the celebrity's vulva. This is problematic for a couple of reasons. First, it is clearly insulting to the women whose vulvas are being commented on. Secondly, and perhaps more importantly considering that celebrities are less likely to read the commentary, someone without prior vulva knowledge may use these images and corresponding comments to make assumptions about their own genitalia. Somewhere out there may be a young woman who is reading about her favorite pop-star or socialite, and then gets a sense from the comments that vulvas should always be perfectly waxed or always have short or long labia and so on. Young women have enough to worry about. Do we really need to suggest that women are to be judged by their genitals, too?

THE DOWN THERE UPSIDE

Fortunately, not all technology has led to vulva-negative outcomes. In fact, we think that technological advances have led to positive vulva developments, as well. First of all, the Internet can be a great way to meet people who share an interest in vulva promotion/advocacy. You

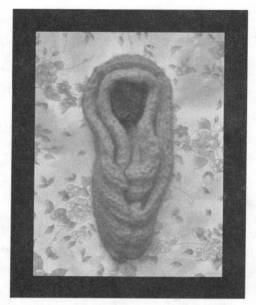

Knit Vulva from the International Vulva Knitting Circle Collection
(Image © Rachel Liebert, Founder of the International Vulva Knitting Circle.)

can see a list of some web sites and communities that we love (including our own podcast *Genitales*—a shameless plug, we know) in the Resources section. As you can probably tell from the craft projects included in this book, we believe that vulva craft is a great form of activism in addition to being a heck of a lot of fun. One of our favorite genital crafters is Rachel Leibert, founder of the International Vulva Knitting Circle.

VULVA ARTS AND CRAFTS

If you are not much of a knitter but still support or love vulva arts and crafts, the Internet has made it possible for you to easily own a variety of vulva products. You can get everything from sofas to lip-balms to jewelry to bicycle covers shaped like vulvas (see Resources).

AN INTERVIEW WITH THE FOUNDER OF THE INTERNATIONAL VULVA KNITTING CIRCLE, RACHEL LIEBERT

"The International Vulva Knitting Circle was founded in 2008 as a grass-roots activist collective in support of The New View campaign's WTF-ing against the emerging industry of female genital cosmetic surgeries. We wanted to mass-produce our own line of diverse lady-bits to speak back to the increasing ways in which female bodies and sexualities are colonized by corporate practices. Within a year we had nearly 150 deliciously different vulvas from people across eleven cities and five countries, and over 500 members of all ages, genders, and geographies.

"People either craft on their own or host circles, although politically we prefer the latter as it more so spoons the dialogue and solidarity needed for broader social change. Either way, we discourage the use [of] patterns (diversity!) so long as people include the labia majora, the labia minora, and of course Her Highness the Clitoris. All skill-levels and crafts are welcomed.

"Late 2009 our first public exhibition was held in Brooklyn, NYC, at a grass-roots event called Vulvagraphics, which pulled together the work of a number of artists celebrating female genital diversity. This event launched the International Vulva Knitting Circle as a traveling exhibition to support localized activism in different parts of the world. We only ask that with any event, it remains grass-roots, fits broadly within our political feminist agenda, and involves people from the community contributing their own crafted vulvas to the traveling collection.

"Our vision is for The Vulva Train to just keep on growing and moving, with women uniquely and collectively crafting resistance to the regulation of their bodies and sexualities.

"And it all begins with the not-so-lady-like knitting needle.

"So, join us!"

Learn more about the International Vulva Knitting Circle in our Resources section.

There is no end to the neat things that one can create to look like or honor a vulva. One of our absolute favorite products is the vulva puppet (the original is called the Wondrous Vulva Puppet and it's made by Dorrie Lane). Vulva puppets come in a variety of shapes, sizes, and materials but typically contain a clitoral hood, a fluffy clitoris, puffy inner and outer labia, a lovely inner lining, and a button or flower urethra and vagina. The best part is that you can stick your hand inside to move the lips of the vulva! The reason we love the vulva puppet so much is because it serves several purposes. Not only is it a great conversation piece as a decoration around your home (or in our case, our offices), but it is also a wonderful tool for teaching about the vulva. Even we understand that some people may feel uncomfortable looking at pictures of the vulva, especially if they have never seen one before. Using vulva puppets as sex-education props helps us to quickly and easily explain the parts of the vulva in a nonintimidating way that is easy for anyone to understand, and it is particularly kid-friendly. This was best demonstrated to a national audience when Debby made the vulva puppet famous by bringing it on *The Tyra Banks Show* while explaining the parts of the vulva. That's right: Debby's vulva puppet has met Tyra, not to mention sex columnist and author Dan Savage, who graciously slipped his hand into her vulva puppet. (If he denies it, remind him that we have photographic evidence.)

Pootie Attack

Sadly, not everyone shares our love for vulva arts and crafts. For instance, two vulva crafters recently ran into some major issues on a popular web site designed to sell homemade crafts. Prior to these issues, the web site was a major source of revenue for these crafters and was one of the best ways for them to sell crafts on the web. However, both ran into resistance from the web site and beyond. The web site prohibited the crafters from tagging their products with certain names such as "feminist" that helped to drive their business. It also

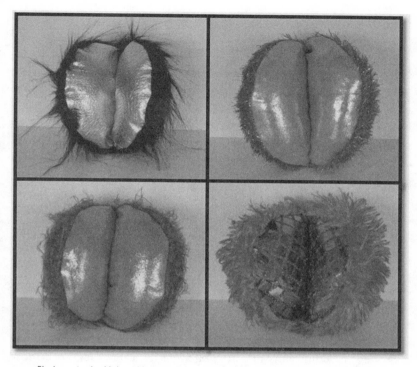

Plushpooties by Melissa Nannen. From left to right: Gilded Pussy, Everybody Loves a Redhead Pussy, Marge Simpson's Pussy, Lucille Ball Disco Pussy (© Melissa Nannen. See more of her work at www.MelissaNannen.com.)

asked them to label their materials as "mature" or "explicit" despite the fact that many of these crafts were simply symbolic representations of vulvas and were not sexualized in any way.

Beyond the web site, a counter web site designed to mock the crafts of the original site targeted the vulva crafters specifically. The vulva crafters felt mocked and discouraged. Melissa Nannen, a friend of Vanessa's who creates Plushpooties (simple vulvas of various colors and sizes with pubic hair shells that are often joyfully comical in appearance and name), removed her pooties from the web site after an attack on one of her art pieces. She wrote on her blog that she was hurt by it because the comments "were much more concerned with the type of person who made them rather than the object itself."[24] That's the strange thing about vulva craft, art, or even research. All too often, assumptions are made about the behaviors and attitudes of those who create or conduct it. We know that these critiques come with the job, but sometimes when we tell people what we do, it is hard to ignore the fact that they are going into TSA scanner mode, wondering what is up with us down there. We try our best to use these responses as fuel for our fire. After all, talking about the vulva is only strange if no one else does it!

As vulva researchers, artists, authors, and crafters, we are opening ourselves up to people who are critical of the vulva, but what really gets our muffs mad is when the vulva itself is attacked. Take for instance a recent celebrity blogger with a huge following who posted an image of several lovely vulva necklaces for sale. These particular necklaces came in several shapes and sizes, and the designs were based on images of real women's vulvas. The blog about the necklaces was sarcastic and critical of the idea of vulva necklaces, but the blogger did not attack the actual appearance of the necklaces. The viewers' comments on the blog were another story, with most comments containing a variation of "ewwww" or "gross." Several comments attacked the appearance of specific vulva pieces, including one web site commentator who said, "The black one looks like that fake dog chit [*sic*]!!" Another person insulted the appearance of all the vulva necklace models by saying, "if you have major nasty beefcurtains [*sic*], why the hell would you want to show it off in the first place?? So gross."

Comments like these make us feel sad. While someone probably wrote these comments without thinking twice about the impression that it would make on those who read them (other than hoping it was funny, perhaps), these comments have the potential to impact women of all ages and all vulva types. Let's say, for example, that you are checking out your favorite celebrity blog when you happen upon a necklace that just happens to look surprisingly similar to your very own lady bits. *Wow*, you think, *how great that someone thought my genitals were beautiful enough to accessorize an outfit!* You feel empowered until you scroll down a bit farther and read the reaction to your genital doppelgangers. Then, you read the series of negative reactions to your "beefcurtains." Sure it's just one little message. However, given that you probably do not come across a mini-version of your muff every day, this feedback may become quite meaningful and even harmful to how you feel about your genitals. So, how do these messages change the way women feel about their genitals, you ask? We cover that (and a whole lot more) in chapter 4.

CUNTCLUSIONS

Vulva art has been around almost as long as vulvas themselves. Vulvas have been portrayed as everything from humorous to dangerous to disgusting. The relatively recent invention of the Internet has exposed us to vulva culture in ways that are continually changing. So what can we do to make sure that change is a positive one?

1. **Support small vulva crafters when you can.** Low on cash? No worries, support does not have to mean financial support these days. Consider "liking" them on Facebook, sharing their craft web sites on your Facebook page (so that friends with cash to spare might support them), or tweeting their web site with a positive message to your friends/followers.

2. **Craft is not just for the crafty!** This book contains tons of tips for fun vulva crafts that you can do yourself or with a group of friends. Instead of a book club (unless, of course, this is the book), consider assembling a vulva-crafting club at your school or in your community.

3. **See a vulva-negative comment on a web site?** Take a minute and post a positive one! It may be your message that makes someone think or feel differently about her vulva.

4. **Keep talking.** Remember when your mother used to say, "If you don't have something nice to say, don't say anything at all"? Well, we disagree. Sometimes even the "not nice" things will get a conversation going. The worst thing that we can do to our vulvas is ignore them. So above all else, let's keep the conversation going!

TEST YOUR VQ

1. What is the first vulva image created by (wo)man?
   a. sheela-na-gig carvings found around Europe
   b. Baubo figurines in Greece
   c. paparazzi shots of young socialites as they exit their limos
   d. *Venus of Willendorf*

2. What is a speculum party?
   a. A pact by women to visit their gynecologists on the same day
   b. When your gynecologist makes a house call
   c. A group of women who examine their own vulvas and vaginas together
   d. the decoration of speculums

3. What is a vulva puppet?
   a. a female puppet with an enlarged vulva
   b. a plushy vulva with a slit in the back for your hand
   c. a BDSM activity
   d. a character created by Jim Henson in the 1950s

Answers

1. d
2. c
3. b

Notes

CHAPTER 1

1. V. Braun and S. Wilkinson, "Socio-Cultural Representations of the Vagina," *Journal of Reproductive and Infant Psychology* 19, no. 1 (2001).

2. C. Blackledge, *The Story of V: A Natural History of Female Sexuality* (New Brunswick, NJ: Rutgers University Press, 2004).

3. A. Kingsley, "A Conference at UNLV Urges Women to Love Their Lady Parts," *Las Vegas: City Life*, September 30, 2010.

4. L. Alptraum, "'Cunts for Fags' Teaches Gay Men How the Other Half Fucks," 2008. http://boinkology.com/2008/02/01/cunts-for-fags-teaches-gay-men-how-the-other-half-fucks. Accessed May 2, 2011.

5. J. Blank, *Femalia* (San Francisco, CA: Down There Press, 1993).

6. B. Dodson, *Sex for One: The Joy of Selfloving* (New York: Crown Trade Paperbacks, 1996).

7. N. Karras, *Petals* (San Diego, CA: Crystal River Publishing, 2003).

8. J. Lloyd, N. S. Crouch, C. L. Minto, L-M Liao, and S. M. Creighton, "Female Genital Appearance: Normality Unfolds," *BJOG: An International Journal of Obstetrics & Gynaecology* 112, no. 5 (2005): 643–46.

9. Betty Dodson, *Viva la Vulva!* (New York: Betty Dodson, 1998).

10. O. Lunde, "A Study of Body Hair Density and Distribution in Normal Women," *American Journal of Physical Anthropology* 64, no. 2 (1984): 179–84.

11. V. Schick, B. N. Rima, and S. K. Calabrese, "Evulvalution: The Portrayal of Women's External Genitalia and Physique Across Time and the Current Barbie Doll Ideals," *The Journal of Sex Research* 48 (2011): 74–81.

12. R. Robinson, *Georgia O'Keeffe: A Life* (Hanover: University Press of New England, 1999).

13. M. Paley, *The Book of the Penis* (New York: Grove Press, 1999).

14. L. M. Liao, L. Michala, and S. M. Creighton, "Labial Surgery for Well Women: A Review of the Literature," *BJOG: An International Journal of Obstetrics and Gynaecology* 117, no. 1 (2010): 20–25.

15. ACOG, "ACOG Committee Opinion No. 378: Vaginal 'Rejuvenation' and Cosmetic Vaginal Procedures," *Obstetrics and Gynecology* 110 (2007): 737–38.

16. J. M. Miklos, "RD Labiaplasty of the Labia Minora: Patients' Indications for Pursuing Surgery," *Journal of Sexual Medicine* 5, no. 6 (2008): 1492–95.

17. V. Braun, "Female Genital Cosmetic Surgery: A Critical Review of Current Knowledge and Contemporary Debates," *Journal of Womens Health* 19, no. 7 (2010): 1393–1407.

18. M. P. Goodman, "Female Cosmetic Genital Surgery," *Obstetrics and Gynecology* 113, no. 2 (2009): 154–59.

19. V. Braun and C. Kitzinger, "'Snatch,' 'Hole,' or 'Honey-pot'? Semantic Categories and the Problem of Nonspecificity in Female Genital Slang," *Journal of Sex Research* 38, no. 2 (2001): 146–58.

20. H. E. O'Connell, J. M. Hutson, C. R. Anderson, & R. J. Plenter, "Anatomical Relationship Between Urethra and Clitoris," *The Journal of Urology* 159, no. 6 (1998): 1892.

21. H. O'Connell and J. O. L. Delancey, "Clitoral Anatomy in Nulliparous, Healthy, Premenopausal Volunteers Using Unenhanced Magnetic Resonance Imaging," *The Journal of Urology* 173, no. 6 (2005): 2060.

22. B. R. Komisaruk, C. Beyer, and B. Whipple, *The Science of Orgasm* (Baltimore, MD: Johns Hopkins University Press, 2006).

23. M. Reece, D. Herbenick, and B. Dodge, "Penile Dimensions and Men's Perceptions of Condom Fit and Feel," *Sexually Transmitted Infections* 85 (2009):127–31.

24. H. Wessells, T. F. Lue, and J. W. McAninch, "Penile Length in Flaccid and Erect States: Guidelines for Penile Augmentation," *Journal of Urology* 156, no. 3 (1996): 995–97.

25. A. K. Ladas, B. Whipple, and J. D. Perry, *The G Spot and Other Recent Discoveries about Human Sexuality* (New York: Holt, Rinehart, and Winston, 1982).

26. A. C. Kinsey, *Sexual Behavior in the Human Female* (Philadelphia, PA: Saunders, 1953).

27. W. H. J. Masters, V. E. Johnson, *Human Sexual Response* (Boston, MA: Little, Brown and Company, 1966).

28. G. L. Gravina, F. Brandetti, P. Martini, E. Carosa, S. M. Di Stasi, S. Morano, A. Lenzi, and E. A. Jannini, "Measurement of the Thickness of the Urethrovaginal Space in Women with or without Vaginal Orgasm," *Journal of Sexual Medicine* 5 (2008): 610–18.

29. A. V. Burri, L. Cherkas, and T. D. Spector, "Genetic and Environmental Influences on Self-Reported G-Spots in Women: A Twin Study," *Journal of Sexual Medicine* 7, no. 5 (2010): 1842–52.

30. D. Herbenick, V. Schick, M. Reece, S. Sanders, B. Dodge, and J. D. Fortenberry, "The Female Genital Self-Image Scale (FGSIS): Results from a Nationally Representative Probability Sample of Women in the United States," *Journal of Sexual Medicine* 8, no. 1 (2011): 158–66.

CHAPTER 2

1. E. G. Stewart and P. Spencer, *The V Book: A Doctor's Guide to Complete Vulvovaginal Health* (New York: Bantam Books, 2002).

2. C. Sonne, "Genital Allergy," *Sexually Transmitted Infections* 80 (2004): 4–7.

3. B. Reed, D. W. Gorenflo, B. W. Gillespie, C. L. Pierson, and P. Zazove, "Sexual Behaviors and Other Risk Factors for Candida Vulvovaginitis," *Journal of Women's Health and Gender Based Medicine* 9, no. 6 (2000): 645–56.

4. J. Todd, "Toxic Shock Syndrome—Evolution of an Emerging Disease," *Advances in Experimental Medicine and Biology* 697 (2011): 175–81.

5. A. E. Hochwalt, M. B. Jones, and S. J. Meyer, "Clinical Safety Assessment of an Ultra Absorbency Menstrual Tampon," *Journal of Women's Health* 19, no. 2 (2010): 273–78.

6. "Tampons and Asbestos, Dioxin and Toxic Shock Syndrome," 2009, http://www.fda.gov/MedicalDevices/Safety/AlertsandNotices/PatientAlerts/ucm070003htm.

7. M. Guida, A. D. S. Sardo, S. Bramante, S. Sparice, G. Acunzo, G. A. Tommaselli, C. Di Carlo, M. Pellicano, E. Greco, and C. Nappi, "Effects of

Two Types of Hormonal Contraception—Oral Versus Intravaginal—on the Sexual Life of Women and Their Partners," *Human Reproduction* 20, no. 4 (2005): 1100–1106.

8. S. D. Fihn, R. H. Latham, P. Roberts, K. Running, and W. E. Stamm, "Association between Diaphragm Use and Urinary Tract Infection," *Journal of the American Medical Association* 254 (1985): 240–45.

9. A. K. Leung, W. L. Robson, and J. Tay-Uyboco, "The Incidence of Labial Fusion in Children," *Journal Pediatric Child Health* 29 (1993): 235–36.

10. D. Muram, "Treatment of Prepubertal Girls with Labial Adhesions," *Journal of Pediatric and Adolescent Gynecology* 12, no. 2 (1999): 67–70.

11. L. M. Kumetz, E. H. Quint, S. Fisseha, and Y. R. Smith, "Estrogen Treatment Success in Recurrent and Persistent Labial Agglutination," *Journal of Pediatric and Adolescent Gynecology* 19, no. 6 (2006): 381.

12. M. J. Nurzia, K. M. Eickhorst, M. K. Ankem, and J. G. Barone, "The Surgical Treatment of Labial Adhesions in Pre-pubertal Girls," *Journal of Pediatric and Adolescent Gynecology* 16, no. 1 (2003): 21.

13. J. Someshwar, R. Lutfi, and L. S. Nield, "The Missing 'Bratz' Doll: A Case of Vaginal Foreign Body," *Pediatric Emergency Care* 23, no. 12 (2007): 897–98.

14. J. Huppert, S. Griffeth, L. Breech, and P. Hillard, "Vaginal Burn Injury Due to Alkaline Batteries," *Journal of Pediatric & Adolescent Gynecology* 22, no. 5 (2009): 133–36.

15. K. Y. Yanoh and Y. Yonemura, "Severe Vaginal Ulcerations Secondary to Insertion of an Alkaline Battery," *Journal of Trauma-Injury Infection & Critical Care* 58, no. 2 (2005): 410–12.

16. Centers for Disease Control and Infection, "Bacterial Vaginosis: CDC Fact Sheet," 2010. http://www.cdc.gov/std/bv/stdfact-bacterial-vaginosis.htm. Accessed February 28, 2011.

CHAPTER 3

1. D. Herbenick, M. Reece, V. Schick, S. A. Sanders, B. Dodge, and J. D. Fortenberry, "Sexual Behavior in the United States: Results from a National Probability Sample of Males and Females Ages 14 to 94," *The Journal of Sexual Medicine* 7 supp. 5 (2010): 255–65.

2. H. E. O'Connell, J. M. Hutson, C. R. Anderson, and R. J. Plenter, "Anatomical Relationship Between Urethra and Clitoris," *The Journal of Urology* 159, no. 6 (1998): 1892.

3. H. E. O'Connell and J. O. L. Delancey, "Clitoral Anatomy in Nulliparous, Healthy, Premenopausal Volunteers Using Unenhanced Magnetic Resonance Imaging," *The Journal of Urology* 173, no. 6 (2005): 2060.

4. S. Ramsey, G. Oades, C. Sweeney, and M. Fraser, "Pubic Hair and Sexuality: A Review," *Journal of Sexual Medicine* 6, no. 8 (2009): 2102–10.

5. R. Levin, "The Ins and Outs of Vaginal Lubrication," *Sexual and Relationship Therapy* 18, no. 4 (2003): 509–13.

6. E. G. Stewart and P. Spencer, *The V Book: A Doctor's Guide to Complete Vulvovaginal Health* (New York: Bantam Books, 2002).

7. D. Herbenick, M. Reece, V. Schick, S. A. Sanders, B. Dodge, and J. D. Fortenberry, "An Event-Level Analysis of the Sexual Characteristics and Composition among Adults Ages 18 to 59: Results from a National Probability Sample in the United States," *The Journal of Sexual Medicine* 7 supp. 5 (2010): 346–61.

8. D. Herbenick, M. Reece, D. Hensel, S. Sanders, K. Jozkowski, and J. D. Fortenberry, "Association of Lubricant Use with Women's Sexual Pleasure, Sexual Satisfaction, and Genital Symptoms: A Prospective Daily Diary Study Journal of Sexual Medicine," *Journal of Sexual Medicine* 8, no. 1 (2011): 202–12.

9. C. M. Meston, R. J. Levin, M. L. Sipski, E. M. Hull, and J. R. Heiman, "Women's Orgasm," *Annual Review of Sex Research* 15 (2004): 173–257.

10. B. R. Komisaruk, C. Beyer, and B. Whipple, *The Science of Orgasm* (Baltimore, MD: Johns Hopkins University Press, 2006).

11. E. W. Eichel, J. D. Eichel, and S. Kule, "The Technique of Coital Alignment and Its Relation to Female Orgasmic Response and Simultaneous Orgasm," *Journal of Sex & Marital Therapy* 14, no. 2 (1988): 129–41.

12. E. W. Eichel and P. Nobile, *The Perfect Fit: How to Achieve Mutual Fulfillment and Monogamous Passion through the New Intercourse* (New York: D. I. Fine, 1992).

13. D. F. Hurlbert and C. Apt, "The Coital Alignment Technique and Directed Masturbation: A Comparative Study on Female Orgasm," *Journal of Sex & Marital Therapy* 21, no. 1 (1995): 21.

14. A. Pierce, "The Coital Alignment Technique (CAT): An Overview of Studies," *Journal of Sex and Marital Therapy* 26, no. 3 (2000): 257–68.

15. M. Reece, D. Herbenick, S. A. Sanders, B. Dodge, A. Ghassemi, and J. D. Fortenberry, "Prevalence and Characteristics of Vibrator Use by Men in the United States," *Journal of Sexual Medicine* 6 (2009): 1867–74.

CHAPTER 4

1. M. Reynolds, D. L. Herbenick, and J. H. Bancroft, "The Nature of Childhood Sexual Experiences: Two Studies 50 Years Apart," in *Sexual Development in Childhood*, ed. J. Bancroft (Bloomington: Indiana Indiana University Press, 2003).

2. B. Schuhrke, "Young Children's Curiosity about Other People's Genitals," *Journal of Psychology & Human Sexuality* 12 (2000): 27–48.

3. C. Handler, *Chelsea Chelsea Bang Bang* (New York: Grand Central Pub., 2010).

4. R. Bramwell, "Invisible Labia: The Representation of Female External Genitals in Women's Magazines," *Sexual & Relationship Therapy* 17, no. 2 (2002): 187–90.

5. V. Schick, B. N. Rima, and S. K. Calabrese, "Evulvalution: The Portrayal of Women's External Genitalia and Physique across Time and the Current Barbie Doll Ideals," *The Journal of Sex Research* 48 (2011): 74–81.

6. G. Edgren, *The Playboy Book: Forty Years* (London: Mitchell Beazley, 1994).

7. J. R. Petersen, *The Century of Sex: Playboy's History of the Sexual Revolution, 1900–1999* (New York: Grove Press, 1999).

8. J. Robertson, *50 Years of the Playboy Bunny* (San Francisco, CA: Chronicle Books, 2010).

9. M. Voracek and M. Fisher, "Shapely Centrefolds? Temporal Change in Body Measures: Trend Analysis," *British Medical Journal* 325, no. 7378 (2002): 1447–48.

10. H. Howarth, V. Sommer, and F. M. Jordan, "Visual Depictions of Female Genitalia Differ Depending on Source," *Medical Humanities* 36, no. 2 (2010): 75.

11. N. Karras, *Petals* (San Diego, CA: Crystal River Publishing, 2003).

12. J. Blank, *Femalia* (San Francisco, CA: Down There Press, 1993).

13. V. Schick, S. Calabrese, and B. Rima, "Does (Labia) Size Really Matter? The Distorting Impact of Exposure to Unrealistic Labia Minora Images on Women's Perceived Labia Size: Implications for Genital Discontent and Sexuality," Annual Meeting of Society for the Scientific Study of Sexuality, San Juan, Puerto Rico, 2008.

14. V. Schick, S. K. Calabrese, B. N. Rima, and A. N. Zucker, "Genital Appearance Dissatisfaction: Implications for Women's Genital Image Self-Consciousness, Sexual Esteem, Sexual Satisfaction, and Sexual Risk," *Psychology of Women Quarterly* 34 (2010): 394–404.

15. E. G. Stewart and P. Spencer, *The V Book: A Doctor's Guide to Complete Vulvovaginal Health* (New York: Bantam Books, 2002).

16. M. B. Oscarsson and E. Benzein, "Women's Experience of Pelvic Examination: An Interview Study," *Obstetrics and Gynecology* 23 (2002): 17–25.

17. *Embarrassing Bodies*, http://www.channel4embarrassingillnesses.com. Accessed February 11, 2011.

18. J. Ashton, *Hygeia Gynecology*, http://www.drjenniferashton.com/labiaplasty.asp. Accessed February 26, 2011.

19. M. P. Goodman, "Female Cosmetic Genital Surgery," *Obstetrics and Gynecology* 113, no. 2 (2009): 154–59.

20. V. Braun, "Female Genital Cosmetic Surgery: A Critical Review of Current Knowledge and Contemporary Debates," *Journal of Womens Health* 19, no. 7 (2010): 1393–1407.

21. V. Braun, "In Search of (Better) Sexual Pleasure: Female Genital Cosmetic Surgery," *Sexualities* 8, no. 4 (2005): 407–24.

22. V. Braun, "Selling the Perfect Vulva," in *Cosmetic Surgery: A Feminist Primer*, eds. C. J. Heyes and M. R. Jones (Farnham, Surrey: Ashgate, 2009).

23. V. Braun and L. Tiefer, "The 'Designer Vagina' and the Pathologisation of Female Genital Diversity: Interventions for Change," *Radical Psychology* 8, no. 1 (2009).

24. M. Farage and H. Maibach, "Lifetime Changes in the Vulva and Vagina," *Archives of Gynecology and Obstetrics* 273, no. 4 (2006): 195–202.

25. T. Lewis, "The Lengths We Go for Beauty," *Newsweek*, July 19, 2010.

26. F. J. Green, "From Clitoridectomies to Designer Vaginas: The Medical Construction of Heteronormative Female Bodies and Sexuality through

Female Genital Cutting," *Sexualities Evolution & Gender* 7, no. 2 (2005): 153–87.

27. S. Moore, H. Gridley, K. Taylor, and K. Johnson, "Women's Views about Intimate Examinations and Sexually Inappropriate Practices by Their General Practitioners," *Psychology and Health* 15 (2000): 71–84.

28. R. K. Reinholtz and C. L. Muehlenhard, "Genital Perceptions and Sexual Activity in a College Population," *The Journal of Sex Research* 32, no. 2 (1995): 155–65.

CHAPTER 5

1. B. S. Czerwinski, "Clinical Studies—Variation in Feminine Hygiene Practices as a Function of Age," *Journal of Obstetric, Gynecologic, and Neonatal Nursing* 29, no. 6 (2000).

2. S. J. Emans, E. R. Woods, E. N. Allred, and E. Grace, "Hymenal Findings in Adolescent Women: Impact of Tampon Use and Consensual Sexual Activity," *The Journal of Pediatrics* 125, no. 1 (1994): 153–60.

3. K. Stewart, M. Powell, and R. Greer, "An Alternative to Conventional Sanitary Protection: Would Women Use a Menstrual Cup?" *Journal of Obstetrics and Gynaecology* 29, no. 1 (2009): 49–52.

4. D. Merskin, "Adolescence, Advertising, and the Ideology of Menstruation," *Sex Roles* 40 (1999): 941.

5. M. Simes and D. H. Berg, "Surreptitious Learning: Menarche and Menstrual Product Advertisements," *Health Care for Women International* 22, no. 5 (2001): 455–69.

6. M. A. Ott, S. Ofner, and J. D. Fortenberry, "Beyond Douching: Use of Feminine Hygiene Products and STI Risk among Young Women," *Journal of Sexual Medicine* 6, no. 5 (2009): 1335–40.

7. R. B. Ness, S. L. Hillier, H. E. Richter, D. E. Soper, C. Stamm, D. C. Bass, R. L. Sweet, and S. Aral, "Why Women Douche and Why They May or May Not Stop," *Sexually Transmitted Diseases* 30, no. 1 (2003): 71–74.

8. J. L. Martino and S. H. Vermund, "Vaginal Douching: Evidence for Risks or Benefits to Women's Health," *Epidemiologic Reviews* 24, no. 3 (2002): 109–24.

9. Instructions, My New Pink Button.

10. W. R. Anderson, D. J. Summerton, D. M. Sharma, and S. A. Holmes, "The Urologist's Guide to Genital Piercing," *BJU International* 91, no. 3 (2003): 245–51.

CHAPTER 6

1. M. Kilmer, "Genital Phobia and Depilation," *Journal of Hellenic Studies* 102 (1982): 104–12.

2. A. Hollander, "The Clothed Image: Picture and Performance," *New Literary History* 1971, no. 2 (1971): 477–93.

3. S. Moalem, *How Sex Works: Why We Look, Smell, Taste, Feel, and Act the Way We Do* (New York: Harper, 2009).

4. S. Ramsey, G. Oades, C. Sweeney, and M. Fraser, "Pubic Hair and Sexuality: A Review," *Journal of Sexual Medicine* 6, no. 8 (2009): 2102–10.

5. J. Chicago, *The Dinner Party: A Symbol of Our Heritage* (Garden City, NY: Anchor Press/Doubleday, 1979).

6. E. Ensler, *The Vagina Monologues* (New York: Villard, 2001).

7. B. Dodson, *Viva la Vulva!* (New York Betty Dodson, 1998).

8. E. G. Stewart and P. Spencer, *The V Book: A Doctor's Guide to Complete Vulvovaginal Health* (New York: Bantam Books, 2002).

9. N. R. Armstrong and J. D. Wilson, "Did the 'Brazilian' Kill the Pubic Louse? *Sexually Transmitted Infections* 82, no. 3 (2006).

10. M. Pale, Sculptures. 2007; http://mimosapale.com/?s=sculptures.

11. A. Kingsley, "A Conference at UNLV Urges Women to Love Their Lady Parts," *Las Vegas: City Life*, September 30, 2010.

12. D. Herbenick, V. Schick, M. Reece, S. Sanders, and J. D. Fortenberry, "Pubic Hair Removal among Women in the United States: Prevalence, Methods and Characteristics," *The Journal of Sexual Medicine* 7, no. 10 (2010): 3322–30.

13. C. Zinko, "Who Needs a Facial When You Can Get a 'Vajacial'?" *San Francisco Chronicle*, June 3, 2010.

14. E. J. Kovavisarach and P. Jirasettasiri, "Randomised Controlled Trial of Perineal Shaving versus Hair Cutting in Parturients on Admission in Labor," *Journal of the Medical Association of Thailand* 88, no. 9 (2005): 1167–71.

CHAPTER 7

1. G. Eknoyan, "A History of Obesity, or How What Was Good Became Ugly and Then Bad," *Advances in Chronic Kidney Disease* 13, no. 4 (2006): 421–27.

2. M. Kohen, "The Venus of Willendorf," *American Imago: A Psychoanalytic Journal for the Arts and Sciences* 3, no. 4 (1946): 49–60.

3. Z. Bahrani, *Women of Babylon: Gender and Representation in Mesopotamia* (London: Routledge, 2001).

4. "Madison Police Blame Halloween Riot on Female Flashers," *Milwaukee News*, November 4, 2002.

5. E. Morris, "Sacred and Obscene Laughter in the Contendings of Horus and Seth, in Egyptian Inversions of Everyday Life, and in the Context of Cultic Competition," in *Egyptian Stories: A British Egyptological Tribute to Alan B Lloyd on the Occasion of his Retirement*, ed. T. S. Schneider and K. Szpakowska (Münster: Ugarit-Verlag, 2007).

6. N. A. Georgopoulos, G. A. Vagenakis, and A. L. Pierris, "Baubo: A Case of Ambiguous Genitalia in the Eleusinian Mysteries," *Hormones* 2, no. 1 (2003): 72–75.

7. M. Marcovich, "Demeter, Baubo, Iacchus, and a Redactor," *Vigiliae Christianae* 40 (1986): 294–301.

8. A. Pearson, "Reclaiming the Sheela-na-gigs: Goddess Imagery in Medieval Sculptures in Ireland," *Canadian Woman Studies* 17, no. 3 (1997): 20–25.

9. H. Ludgate, *London Laid Bare* (Cambridge: Vanguard, 2007).

10. G. Dines, J. M. Humez, and C. G. Aleman, "Gender, Race, and Class in Media: A Text-Reader," *Contemporary Psychology* 41, no. 4 (1996).

11. S. Qureshi, "Displaying Sara Baartman, the 'Hottentot Venus,'" *History of Science* 42 (2004): 233–57.

12. E. Alexander, "The Venus Hottentot (1825)," *Callaloo* 24, no. 3 (2001): 688–91.

13. S. Freud, "Female Sexuality," *International Journal of Psycho-Analysis* 13 (1932): 281–97.

14. C. C. Eldredge, *Georgia O'Keeffe: American and Modern* (New Haven: Yale University Press, 1993).

15. R. Robinson, *Georgia O'Keeffe: A Life* (Hanover: University Press of New England, 1999), 282.

16. J. Chicago, *The Dinner Party: A Symbol of Our Heritage* (Garden City, NY: Anchor Press/Doubleday, 1979).

17. B. Dodson, *Sex for One: The Joy of Selfloving* (New York: Crown Trade Paperbacks, 1996).

18. A. Sprinkle, "Post-Porn Modernist," http://anniesprinkle.org/past/ppm-bobsart/script.html. Accessed February 20, 2011.

19. T. Gomi, *Everyone Poops* (Brooklyn, NY: Kane/Miller Book Publishers, 1993).

20. T. Kapsalis, *Public Privates: Performing Gynecology from Both Ends of the Speculum* (Durham, NC: Duke University Press, 1997).

21. E. Ensler, *The Vagina Monologues* (New York: Villard, 2001).

22. N. Toubia, "Female Circumcision as a Public Health Issue," *New England Journal of Medicine* 331, no. 11 (1994): 712–16.

23. B. Dodson, "Betty's Response to the Vagina Monologues," http://dodsonandross.com/sexfeature/bettys-response-vagina-monologues. Accessed May 02, 2011.

24. M. Nannen, "Closing Down Plushpootie," http://goodmarvin.blogspot.com/2010/08/closing-down-plushpootie.html. Accessed August 23, 2010.

Resources

TO BROWSE, BUY, OR BORROW

To Read and to Watch: Vulva Visuals

Femalia

In 1993, Joani Blank published a beautiful book full of close-up color images of the vulva, which—at the time of this writing—is sadly out of print. However, it should be back in print from another publisher soon.

> J. Blank. *Femalia*. San Francisco, CA: Down There Press, 1993.
> J. Blank. *Femalia*. San Francisco, CA: Last Gasp, 2010.
> Web: www.joaniblank.com

Petals

Husband-and-wife team Nick and Sayaka Karras published *Petals* in 2003. The lovely coffee table book features a wide variety of vulva images displayed in sepia tones. We met them at a vulva conference in Las Vegas in fall 2010 where they were recruiting volunteers to model for their new book of vulva images. The much-anticipated new book will contain full-color images. Information about their upcoming book, exam-room poster project, and other products are on their web site (www.nickkarras.com).

> N. Karras. *Petals*. San Diego, CA: Crystal River Publishing, 2003.

N. Karras and B. Peacock. *Petals: A Journey into Self-Discovery.* Video (the making of the book). Berlin: Rogner & Bernhard, 2010.

Cunt Coloring Book: Drawings

Although there are no vulva photographs in the *Cunt Coloring Book*, there is a diverse range of vulva drawings. We think that the book is a lot of fun and a great way to open dialogue about genital diversity.

T. Corinne. *Cunt Coloring Book: Drawings.* San Francisco, CA: Last Gasp, 1988.

Body Drama: Real Girls, Real Bodies, Real Issues, Real Answers

Although this is a great book for everybody (complete with pictures of women of many body types), this book is particularly suited for young women. Author Nancy Redd fought to include vulva images in the book, and we praise her for that.

N. Redd. *Body Drama: Real Girls, Real Bodies, Real Issues, Real Answers.* New York: Gotham Books, 2007.

Annie Sprinkle

If we wanted to list every video with images of vulvas in it, we wouldn't have room for anything else. However, we made an exception for Annie Sprinkle's videos. These are not pornography; they celebrate the diversity of women's genitals—and we wanted to celebrate Annie.

J. Kramer and A. Sprinkle. *Fire in the Valley: Female Genital Massage.* Oakland, CA: New School of Erotic Touch, 2004.
A. Sprinkle and J. Kramer. *Zen Pussy: A Meditation on Eleven Vulvas.* Oakland, CA: EroSpirit Research Institute, 1999.
Web: www.anniesprinkle.org

Vulva Health (General)

The V Book: A Doctor's Guide to Complete Vulvovaginal Health

The V Book is one of our favorites, and it's packed with illuminating and easy-to-understand information.

E. G. Stewart and P. Spencer. *The V Book: A Doctor's Guide to Complete Vulvovaginal Health.* New York: Bantam Books, 2002. Web: www.thevbook.com

Vaginas: An Owner's Manual

A book about the vulva from an OB/GYN mother and her daughter.

C. Livoti and E. Topp. *Vaginas: An Owner's Manual.* New York: Thunder's Mouth Press, 2004.

Vulva Culture

Cunt: A Declaration of Independence

Personal vulva stories sprinkled with facts and filled with empowerment.

I. Muscio. *Cunt: A Declaration of Independence.* Seattle: Seal Press, 2002.

Public Privates

Although vulvas may not play the lead, they do a great job in their supporting role in Kapsalis's interesting analysis of the gynecological exam.

T. Kapsalis. *Public Privates: Performing Gynecology from Both Ends of the Speculum.* Durham, NC: Duke University Press, 1997.

Betty's Work

Betty Dodson has produced a range of important work related to women's bodies and sexuality. Among our favorites:

B. Dodson. *Sex for One: The Joy of Selfloving.* New York: Crown Trade Paperbacks, 1996.

B. Dodson. *Orgasms for Two: The Joy of Partnersex.* New York: Harmony, 2002.

B. Dodson. *Celebrating Orgasm: Women's Private Selfloving Sessions.* Video. New York: Betty Dodson, 1996.

B. Dodson. *Viva la Vulva!* Video. New York: Betty Dodson, 1998.

B. Dodson. *Orgasmic Women: 13 Selfloving Divas.* Video. New York: Betty Dodson, 2005.

B. Dodson, K. Decosterd, and ITC Communications. *Selfloving*. Video. New York: Betty Dodson, 1991.

The Dinner Party

Invited to a dinner party with some fabulous women? Forgo the wine and consider this interesting hostess gift instead.

J. Chicago. *The Dinner Party: A Symbol of Our Heritage*. Garden City, NY: Anchor Press/Doubleday, 1979.

The Story of V: A Natural History of Female Sexuality

Coochie culture at its best.

C. Blackledge. *The Story of V: A Natural History of Female Sexuality*. New Brunswick, NJ: Rutgers University Press, 2004.

The Vagina Monologues

This series of monologues by Eve Ensler popularized vagina love.

E. Ensler. *The Vagina Monologues*. New York: Villard, 2001.
E. Ensler. *The Vagina Monologues*. Video. New York, NY: HBO Home Video, 2002.
Web: www.vday.org

OUR CHANGING BODIES

General Health

Our Bodies, Ourselves

A book by women, for women. There are now many editions on numerous relevant topics. All are highly recommended.

Boston Women's Health Book Collective. *Our Bodies, Ourselves: A New Edition for a New Era*. New York: Simon & Schuster, 2005.

Puberty and Your Period

Get a little help navigating those tricky topics with some of these parent-approved titles:

K. Gravelle, J. Gravelle, and D. Palen. *The Period Book: Everything You Don't Want to Ask (But Need to Know).* New York: Walker & Co, 1996.

M. Jukes and D. Tilley. *Growing Up: It's a Girl Thing: Straight Talk about First Bras, First Periods, and Your Changing Body.* New York: Alfred A. Knopf, 1998.

J. A. Loulan, B. Worthen, C. W. Dyrud, and M. Quackenbush. *Period: A Girl's Guide to Menstruation with a Parent's Guide.* Minnetonka, MN: Book Peddlers, 2001.

A. B. Middleman, K. G. Pfeifer, and American Medical Association. *American Medical Association Girl's Guide to Becoming a Teen.* San Francisco, CA: Jossey-Bass, 2006.

P. Schwartz and D. Cappello. *Ten Talks Parents Must Have with Their Children about Sex and Character.* New York: Hyperion, 2000.

Pregnancy

Boston Women's Health Book Collective. *Our Bodies, Ourselves: Pregnancy and Birth.* New York: Touchstone Book/Simon & Schuster, 2008.

Web: www.ourbodiesourselves.org

Menopause

Boston Women's Health Book Collective. *Our Bodies, Ourselves: Menopause.* New York: Simon & Schuster, 2006.

Web: www.ourbodiesourselves.org

SEX

Although a little older, this book is a classic:

J. Heiman and J. LoPiccolo. *Becoming Orgasmic: A Sexual and Personal Growth Program for Women.* New York: Prentice Hall, 1988.

Does this name look familiar? If you liked this book, chances are you may enjoy Debby's first book:

D. Herbenick. *Because It Feels Good: A Woman's Guide to Sexual Pleasure and Satisfaction.* Emmaus, PA: Rodale, 2009.

A contemporary bestseller, this will guide you (or your partner) through everything cunnilingus:

I. Kerner. *She Comes First: The Thinking Man's Guide to Pleasuring a Woman.* New York: ReganBooks, 2004.

What do you get when you combine a neuroscientist, an endocrinologist, and a sexuality researcher? Answer: A really smart and interesting book about orgasm.

B. R. Komisaruk, C. Beyer, and B. Whipple. *The Science of Orgasm.* Baltimore, MD: Johns Hopkins University Press, 2006.

Groundbreaking, great, and glorious. What else could you want in a book about the G-spot?

A. K. Ladas, B. Whipple, and J. D. Perry. *The G-spot and Other Recent Discoveries about Human Sexuality.* New York: Holt, Rinehart, and Winston, 1982.

Does it exist? This book will answer all your questions, and you'll have fun while it does it.

D. Sundahl. *Female Ejaculation & the G-spot.* London: Fusion, 2004.

PERIOD PRODUCTS

Organic Products

Natracare
All natural and organic products, they have a wide range of tampons and pads to fit everyone's needs.

Web: www.natracare.com
Phone: +44 (0) 117 9823492

Seventh Generation

They use 100 percent organic cotton in their products with mostly recycled content to construct their packaging. They carry both tampons and pads.

Web: www.seventhgeneration.com
Phone: 800.456.1191

Menstrual Cups

The DivaCup

Made of healthcare-grade silicone, this menstrual cup has been around for over thirty-five years and is approved by the FDA.

Web: www.divacup.com
Phone: 866.444.DIVA (3482)

The Keeper

Invented in 1987, the Keeper is FDA approved for its intended use. Although the material is natural (gum rubber), it is not recommended for those with a latex allergy.

Web: www.keeper.com
Phone: 800.500.0077

The Moon Cup

For those with allergies to latex, the Moon Cup is made from medical-grade silicone. Like the other two products, it is FDA approved.

Web: www.mooncup.com
Phone: 800.500.0077

Fabric Pads

Comfy Cloth Pads

They sell a variety of pads, pad bags, pantyliners, and other pad paraphernalia.

Web: www.comfyclothpads.com

Gladrags

A variety of different products to fill all your period needs.

> Web: www.gladrags.com
> Phone: 800.799.4523

Lunapads

A large selection of pads, kits, pantyliners, and even underwear with pads attached.

> Web: www.lunapads.com
> Phone: 888.590.2299

VULVA STUFF(ED)

BadMimi

If loving Mimi is bad, we don't want to be good! Find vulva pillows, pens, and other products.

> Web: www.badmimi.com
> Phone: 707.332.5117

Etsy

Search for everything from artwork to custom vulva pendants to pictures of your poonanny.

> Web: www.etsy.com; popular vulva product sellers: VulvaLoveLovely,
> DeviantCandy, WomaninBloom, ArtbyWinona

Feminist Women's Health Center

They provide two speculum options at good prices: a full kit with a speculum and a speculum (only). In addition to the speculum, the kit includes a mirror, flashlight, lubricant, and instructions. They carry three different sizes: small, medium, and large.

> Web: www.fwhc.org

House O'Chicks
The home of the original Wondrous Vulva Puppet by Dorrie Lane.

Web: www.houseochicks.com

Nutty Tarts
This Finnish team of artists puts the pubes in panties with their hairy underwear collection.

Web: www.nuttytarts.com

Plush Pooties
Our friend makes these neat little pooties that come in fun names like Squirrel and Cookie Monster Pussy.

Web: www.melissanannen.com

Yoni
Your source for everything yoni, including the Wondrous Vulva Puppet!

Web: www.yoni.com

HAIR IT IS

Less

Shave or Trim
You don't need any fancy-schmancy tools for this. A good pair of scissors or a sharp razor/shaving-cream combination should do the trick, but if you are looking for a product that does it all (in the shower), we recommend the Schick Quattro TrimStyle.

Web: www.quattroforwomen.com
Phone: 800.SHAVERS (742.8377)

Electrolysis

If you'd like to say a more permanent good-bye to your pubic hair, you may want to look into electrology. If you do, the American Electrology Association hosts a list of certified electrologists.

Web: www.electrology.com

More

Merkins

You may want to check-in (or merk-in) with your local wig store to ask whether they carry these fun little wigs for wear down there. If not, we found them for order from:

Max Wigs

Web: www.maxwigs.com
Phone: 888.661.8884

International Wigs

Web: www.internationalwig.com
Phone: 800.344.4999

Different

Betty Beauty

Betty Beauty makes dye especially for your hair down there. They come in natural (black, brown, blond, and red) and fun colors (pink, purple, blue, and green). In addition to selling dye, they have stencils and crystal body stickers.

Webs: www.bettybeauty.com
Phone: 888.44.BETTY (23889)

PLACES TO GO, PEOPLE TO SEE, CAUSES TO SUPPORT

Women's Sex Organ-ization-s: Happy and Healthy

American Association of Sexuality Educators, Counselors and Therapists (AASECT)

The title says it all! Have a sexuality question? They have an answer.

Web: www.aasect.org
Phone: 202.449.1099
Address: 1444 I St NW, Suite 700, Washington, DC 20005

American Congress of Obstetricians and Gynecologists

A go-to for everything gynecologist. If you have a question, this is the most reliable place to find an answer. Although geared toward professionals, there is definitely something for everyone on their web site.

Web: www.acog.org
Phone: 202.638.5577
Address: PO Box 96920, Washington, DC 20090-6920

American Psychological Association

Find psychologists, support groups, or just general information about anything and everything related to psychology.

Web: www.apa.org
Phone: 800.374.2721
Address: 750 First St NE, Washington, DC 20002-4242

American Social Health Association (ASHA)

Information, referrals, and support groups related to sexually transmitted infections.

Web: www.ashastd.org
Phone: 919.361.8400
Address: PO Box 13827, Research Triangle Park, Durham, NC 27709

Gynecologic Cancer Foundation

Information and referrals related to gynecologic cancers.

Web: www.thegcf.org
Phone: 312.578.1439
Address: 230 W. Monroe, Suite 2528, Chicago, IL 60606

The International Society for the Study of Vulvovaginal Disease

We are both proud members of this vulvologist society. A credible source for cutting-edge vulva research. Contact them to find a medical provider in your area, or browse their web site for patient-education materials.

Web: www.issvd.org
Phone: 704.814.9493
Address: 8814 Peppergrass Ln, Waxhaw, NC 28173

Planned Parenthood

Planned Parenthood has been helping women keep their vulvas happy and healthy for over ninety years. With over 820 health centers across the United States, you can likely find low-cost GYN exams, testing, and birth control at a Planned Parenthood near you.

Web: www.plannedparenthood.org
Phone: 800.230.PLAN (7526)
Address: 434 West 33rd St, New York, NY 10001

National Lichen Sclerosus Support Group (NLSSG)

Based in the United Kingdom (and founded by Fabia Bracken-bury, who also originally dedicated March as Vulval Health Awareness Month), the NLSSG provides information, support, and referrals related to lichen sclerosus, a skin condition that can affect the genitals.

Web: www.lichensclerosus.org

National Vulvodynia Association (NVA)

Provides information related to vulvodynia (vulvar pain), referrals, and newsletters for patients and providers. The NVA is also a source for patient advocacy and research support.

Web: www.nva.org
Phone: 301.299.3999
Address: PO Box 4491, Silver Spring, MD 20914-4491

Sexuality Information and Education Council of the United States

Web: www.siecus.org
Phone: 212.819.9770 (NY)/202.462.2340 (DC)
Addresses: 90 John St, Suite 402, New York, NY 10038
    1706 R Street NW, Washington, DC 20009

Vulval Health Awareness Campaign

Provides information and support related to vulval health conditions. Vulval Health Awareness Month was also founded as part of the campaign.

Phone: +44 07765 947599
Web: www.vhac.org

Vulval Pain Society

Provides information and education about vulval pain to women and their partners. Based in the United Kingdom.

Web: www.vulvalpainsociety.org
Address: PO Box 7804, Nottingham NG3 5ZQ, United Kingdom

Centers of Our Yoni-verse

Center for Sex and Culture

A safe space for sexual education regardless of your sex or gender. If you are ever in the area, they have great workshops including "Cunts for Fags."

Web: www.sexandculture.org
Phone: 415.255.1155
Address: 2261 Market St, Box 455-A, San Francisco, CA 94114

Center for Sexual Health & Pleasure

Sex Ed isn't just for kids! Drop-in for a one-on-one consultation with Ms. Andelloux.

Web: www.thecsph.org
Phone: 401.345.8685
Address: 250 Main St, The Grant Building, Pawtucket RI, 02860

Center for Sexual Health Promotion

Visit our Center's web site to get the latest updates on our research.

Web: www.sexualhealth.indiana.edu
Phone: 812.855.0861
Address: HPER 116, Indiana University, Bloomington, IN 47405

Center for Young Women's Health

A collaboration between the Division of Adolescent & Young Adult Medicine and the Division of Gynecology at Children's Hospital Boston, it is a great place for teens and parents to learn about their changing health needs. Full of great fact sheets, including information about labial adhesions.

Web: www.youngwomenshealth.org
Phone: 617.355.2994
Address: 333 Longwood Ave, 5th fl., Boston, MA 02115

The Kinsey Institute

The one that started it all. We are proud to be associated with The Kinsey Institute, a continued source of research and art about sex and sexuality.

Web: www.kinseyinstitute.org and www.kinseyconfidential.org (for Q&A)
Phone: 812.855.7686
Address: Morrison Hall 313, 1165 E. Third St, Bloomington, IN 47405

Just Causes

The International Vulva Knitting Circle

We said it before and we'll say it again, we love the message of the Circle! Celebrating vulva diversity while doing crafts = a perfect afternoon.

Join/Like them on Facebook: International Vulva Knitting Circle

The Muffia

Sinead King and Katie O'Brien take their muffs to the streets. Outrageously phenomenal performance street artists, they make people stop and think about the ways in which we critique women's bodies.

Web: www.themuffia.co.uk

The New View Campaign

Vulvactivists unite! Originally started to challenge Female Sexual Dysfunction in 2000, they now have a variety of pro-genital programs successfully connecting academics and activists.

Web: www.newviewcampaign.org
Address: PO Box 1845, New York, NY 10159-1845

Pads4Girls

Girls in developing countries may be forced to miss school or work if they do not have the proper tools (e.g., tampons, pads) to help them manage their periods. Pads4Girls donates reusable pads to women and girls in need through several different programs listed on their web site. They will take cash or pad donations!

Web: www.lunapads.com/padsfgirls

V-Day

It all began with a single performance of *The Vagina Monologues*. This past year, there were over fifty-four hundred events (including performances of *The Vagina Monologues*) to raise money and awareness to end violence against women and girls globally.

Web: www.vday.org
Phone: 212.645.8329

Female-Friendly Sex Shops (listed alphabetically)

Ann Summers

Web: www.annsummers.com
Phone: +44 0845 456 6948
Multiple locations across the UK. In-home parties.

Aphrodite's Toy Box

Web: www.aphroditestoybox.com
Phone: 404.292.9700
Address: 3040 N. Decatur Rd, Atlanta, GA 30079

Babeland

Web: www.babeland.com
Phone: 800.658.9119
Addresses:
  707 E. Pike St, Seattle, WA 98122
  462 Bergen St (Flatbush/5th Ave), Brooklyn, NY 11217
  94 Rivington St (Ludlow/Orchard), New York, NY 10002
  43 Mercer St (Broome/Grand), New York, NY 10013

Early to Bed

Web: www.early2bed.com
Phone: 866.585.2BED (2233)
Address: 5232 N. Sheridan Rd, Chicago, IL 60640

For Your Pleasure

Web: www.foryourpleasure.com
Phone: 603.925.4397
In-home parties throughout the United States and Canada

Good for Her

Web: www.goodforher.com
Phone: 877.588.0900
Address: 175 Harbord St, Toronto, Canada M5S 1H3

Good Vibrations

Web: www.goodvibes.com
Phone: 800.BUY.VIBE (289.8423)
Locations:
    899 Mission St, San Francisco, CA 94103
    603 Valencia St, San Francisco, CA 94110
    1620 Polk St, San Francisco, CA 94109
    2504 San Pablo Ave, Berkeley, CA 94702
    308A Harvard St, Brookline, MA 02446

My Pleasure

Web: www.mypleasure.com
Phone: 866.697.5327

NOMIA

Web: www.nomiaboutique.com
Phone: 207.773.4774
Address: 24 Exchange St, Suite 215 (2nd fl.), Portland, ME 04101

Passion Parties

Web: www.passionparties.com
Phone: 800.4.PASSION (727.7466)
In-home parties throughout the United States and Canada

Pure Romance

Web: www.pureromance.com
Phone: 866.ROMANCE (766.2623)
In-home parties throughout the United States and Puerto Rico (and expanding!)

Self Serve Toys

Web: www.selfservetoys.com
Phone: 505.265.5815
Address: 3904B Central Ave SE, Albuquerque, NM 87108

She Bop

Web: www.sheboptheshop.com
Phone: 503.473.8018
Address: 909 N. Beech St, Portland, OR 97227

Smitten Kitten

Web: www.smittenkittenonline.com
Phone: 888.751.0523
Address: 3010 Lyndale Ave S, Minneapolis, MN 55408

Sugar

Web: www.sugartheshop.com
Phone: 410.467.2632
Address: 927 W. 36th St (Hampden), Baltimore, MD

Surprise Parties

Web: www.surpriseparties.com
Phone: 1.877.Surpriz (787.7749)
In-home parties throughout the United States

Tulip Toy Gallery

Web: www.mytulip.com
Phone: 877.70.TULIP (88547)
Locations:
  1422 Milwaukee Ave, Chicago, IL 60622
  3459 N. Halsted St, Chicago, IL 60657
  1480 W. Berwyn Ave, Chicago, IL 60640

Va Va Voom

Web: www.vavavooom.com
Phone: 828.254.6329
Address: 36 Battery Park Ave, Asheville, NC 28801

Whole DC

Web: www.facebook.com/WholeDC
Phone: TBD. Keep an eye out for this LGBT-friendly sex shop.

Index

About the Authors

Debby Herbenick, PhD, is associate director and research scientist at the Center for Sexual Health Promotion, Indiana University; the sexual health educator for the Kinsey Institute for Research in Sex, Gender, and Reproduction; and a widely read sex columnist for various newspapers and magazines. She is also the author of *Because It Feels Good: A Woman's Guide to Sexual Pleasure and Satisfaction* (2009) and the forthcoming *I Love You More Book* (StoryPeople Press). She has served as an expert on the vagina and vulva (and other sex topics) for the *Tyra Banks Show* and *The Doctors* and writes about sex for MySexProfessor.com, *Psychology Today, WebMD,* and *Men's Health* magazine. She is also a member of the International Society for the Study of Vulvovaginal Disease, the International Society for the Study of Women's Sexual Health, and the International Academy of Sex Research. As a widely cited sex expert, she has been quoted in more than five hundred magazine and newspaper articles including those in the *New York Times, LA Times, San Francisco Chronicle, Washington Post, Cosmopolitan, Glamour, Marie Claire, Women's Health, Men's Health,* and *SELF.*

Vanessa Schick, PhD, is a social psychologist and a research scientist at the Center for Sexual Health Promotion, Indiana University. She has conducted a variety of studies on the vulva that have been published in peer-reviewed journals ranging from the changes in the portrayal of the vulva in sexually explicit magazines to understanding how women's concerns about their vulva appearance impact them in the bedroom. She has presented her work to diverse audiences, from the Kinsey Institute to students in the classroom to sex researchers at the European Federation of Sexology conference in Rome, Italy. She is also a member of the International Society for the Study of Vulvo-vaginal Disease and the International Academy of Sex Research.

Dr. Herbenick and Dr. Schick are also two of the scientists be-hind the National Survey of Sexual Health and Behavior (NSSHB), the largest nationally representative study of sexual behavior in the United States, which surveyed individuals ages fourteen to ninety-four about their sexual lives.